"DESTROYED FOR LACK OF KNOWLEDGE

THE ULTIMATE HEALTH & WELLNESS GUIDE FOR THE TWENTY FIRST CENTURY

Order this book online at www.trafford.com/08-0001
or email orders@trafford.com

Most Trafford titles are also available at major online book retailers.

© Copyright 2008 Tom Pritchard.
All rights reserved. No part of this publication may be reproduced, stored in a retrieval system, or transmitted, in any form or by any means, electronic, mechanical, photocopying, recording, or otherwise, without the written prior permission of the author.

Note for Librarians: A cataloguing record for this book is available from Library and Archives Canada at www.collectionscanada.ca/amicus/index-e.html

Printed in Victoria, BC, Canada.

ISBN: 978-1-4251-6780-6

We at Trafford believe that it is the responsibility of us all, as both individuals and corporations, to make choices that are environmentally and socially sound. You, in turn, are supporting this responsible conduct each time you purchase a Trafford book, or make use of our publishing services. To find out how you are helping, please visit www.trafford.com/responsiblepublishing.html

Our mission is to efficiently provide the world's finest, most comprehensive book publishing service, enabling every author to experience success. To find out how to publish your book, your way, and have it available worldwide, visit us online at www.trafford.com/10510

Trafford PUBLISHING www.trafford.com

North America & international
toll-free: 1 888 232 4444 (USA & Canada)
phone: 250 383 6864 ♦ fax: 250 383 6804 ♦ email: info@trafford.com

The United Kingdom & Europe
phone: +44 (0)1865 722 113 ♦ local rate: 0845 230 9501
facsimile: +44 (0)1865 722 868 ♦ email: info.uk@trafford.com

10 9 8 7 6 5 4 3 2 1

I have deemed it necessary in the light of the complex subject matter of this book to include a joint foreward by two eminent men ,renowned experts in their own field of expertise.

FOREWARD

Pastor F.J.Turley, General Secretary/Treasurer United Pentecostal Church, Great Britain & Ireland

Reading through this treatise has been a pleasure, & I must confess very illuminating, it is obvious that the author has painstakingly undertaken an in-depth study of the subject in hand & what he has written if taken on board will prove of great value to those who read & apply it.

In recent times the subject of obesity has been very much in the public domain & even the Government health department has issued guidelines concerning it, the media through the various newspapers & periodicals have also highlighted the need for people to address the situation, & especially the younger generation who seem to be hooked on "Junk food".

In view of this lots of schools are now catering for their pupils with more wholesome meals, this is good, parents should also take note of what their children are eating.

Tom has gone into great detail on the matter of Vaccines, Antibiotics, & other medical & Vitamin remedies & those reading this book will benefit if they follow his instructions.

Obviously, in order to enjoy reasonably good health the Laws given by God in the Old Testament to his people if applied today will likewise ensure his blessing.

The Lord who created us certainly knows what is best for us & compliance with his Food Laws can only be to our Physical & Spiritual good.

I was very impressed with the author's treatment of the subject of Divine healing in chapter 8, it was a very balanced & Scriptural presentation of the teaching in view of the distorted presentation given by some Preachers & Evangelists.

The Lord Jesus on the cross paid the price for our sins, therefore as Paul says in 1Cor.6..19-20 "We are bought with a price therefore we are to glorify God in our Bodies & Spirits which are his for our Bodies are the Temple of the Holy Ghost & we are not our own", This surely should be sufficient for us to obey the Food laws of God so that we can be the best we can be for God, to use us & make our bodies his earthly dwelling place.

I trust & pray that this book will have the widest circulation possible so that all the good advice will reach many who are in need of it.

Yours sincerely

F.J.Turley

FORWARD

Doctor Francisco Contreras, Medical Director, Oasis of hope Hospital, Tijuana, Mexico.

How wonderful it is to know that we were not put on this earth to fend for ourselves. In fact, we were wonderfully and fearfully made, and we were left with a magnificent instruction book. "God's instruction book for life" could be a modern day title for the Bible, that is exactly what it is; and one of life's most important subjects is the human body. In all my years of practice, I have absolutely no doubt that what we eat is directly correlated with our health. "You are what you eat", everybody has heard this phrase at least once in their lifetime, it's a phrase that is often thrown around loosely. But do people really know what it means? This phrase may sound like a newly found piece of scientific information but it has been around for thousands of years. We can even quote the illustrious philosopher Hippocrates "Let your food be your medicine and your medicine be your food". Hippocrates must have been in tune with God's instruction book, for this is exactly what God says.

In working with thousands of patients as a surgical oncologist, I have seen first hand how a nutritiously charged diet can help heal the human body, and certainly there are countless scientific studies that prove this. However, the significance of living a nutritious lifestyle is that it's a mandate that comes directly from God. This is the best time to understand the concept of nutrition and embrace it. Everyday we see on the news how massive resources are put into research to find cures for the most deadly diseases, big companies trying desperately to find the elusive silver bullet, in particular for cancer. The truth is there is no silver bullet. A cancerous tumor is merely the symptom of a greater problem. It's clear today that superior doctors, superb equipment, and the latest medications are sometimes not enough. Our entire lifestyle is what can lead us into disease or allow us to come out of it. More importantly the way we live our lives can prevent us from getting sick; this is why prevention is key.

Currently, there is a vast amount of misinformation regarding health, people don't know who or what to believe anymore. The need for a book that provides up-to-date information and more importantly information based on God's principles is vital in the world today. People *need* to know, the title of the book expresses this clearly "Destroyed, for lack of knowledge". What a true and sorrowful statement this can become if we don't change the way we live. It is only if we are properly informed that we can make the decision to change and live a longer, healthier life. Tom Pritchard has skillfully provided this information and gives people the opportunity to change their lifestyle, improve their eating habits, and more importantly follow God's word. "Destroyed, for lack of knowledge" is the perfect starting point to achieve one of the many goals that God has set for us. It is filled with practical, straightforward, and valuable information. Tom Pritchard writes passionately about God's purpose for our health. One can only hope that we can all attain this passion to maintain our bodies in tune with God's plan.

Ultimately, we all live under the grace of God, and only he can decide what our purpose will be here on this earth. But he has left us with an instruction book, in which he has promised to guide us through every aspect of our lives, including how we treat the body that he has given us. We must always be obedient of God's word; this is why this book is an important tool to comply with yet another of God's statutes.

Francisco Contreras, MD

"IN TIMES OF UNIVERSAL DECEIT TELLING THE TRUTH BECOMES A REVOLUTIONARY ACT"
GEORGE ORWELL

CONTENTS

	FOREWARD	3
	FORWARD	6
	PREFACE	12
1	THE LAWS OF GOD	18
2	THE LAW OF CAUSE & EFFECT	24
3	THE BASICS OF THE FOOD LAWS	32
4	THE PURPOSE OF THE FOOD LAWS	39
5	THE RELEVANCE OF THE FOOD LAWS	42
6	THE RELEVANCE OF THE FOOD LAWS TO INDUSTRY	50
7	THE RELEVANCE OF THE FOOD LAWS TO THE INDIVIDUAL	52
8	THE CHRISTIAN & HEALING	59
9	BODY SYSTEMS	64
10	VACCINES	71
11	VITAMINS & DISEASE	81
12	GLUTTONY, THE COMMONEST SIN	106
13	THE UNCLEAN MEATS	115

14	SOME OBJECTIONS	120
15	THE EATING OF BLOOD	122
16	THE EATING OF FAT.	127
17	OUR FURRY FRIENDS	131
18	NATURES REMEDIES	135
19	THE DANGERS OF WHITE SUGAR	144
20 (A)	SACCHARIN (known as "The Pink" because of its wrapper)	147
20 (B)	ASPARTAME (known as "The Blue" because of its wrapper)	149
21	THE AMAZING BENEFITS OF FISH OIL	151
22	PHYSICAL FITNESS	154
23	STRESS!!! A COMMON KILLER	160
24	FEAR & WORRY	165
25	THE DEMON DRINK	169
26	45 FOODS RICH IN VITAMIN B 17	178
27	EIGHT OF THE MOST POTENT IMMUNE SYSTEM BOOSTERS, ALSO VERY HIGH IN ANTI-OXIDANTS, NATURES OWN ANTI-BIOTICS.	182
28	DISEASE CONTROL & SANITATION	183
29	THE DIETARY PROCESS OF WEIGHT REDUCTION	189
30	THEORY & PRACTICE OF DETOXING	194
	EPILOGUE	198
	BIBLIOGRAPHY	203

PREFACE

I was uncertain as to wether or not I should write this book seeing as there have been many books of this nature written before, but the more I thought about it & the more I looked around me the more I became convinced that another book of this nature should be written, only quite differently & in more detail, The Dietary Laws(or Food Laws) of God apply equally to the non Christian as well as the Christian, because the benefits of these Laws of God are available to anyone who has the good sense to follow them, be they Christian or otherwise, indeed many Muslim & Jewish communities have adhered to these principles for centuries & know the benefits of them & many remote tribes of the worlds rain forests have lived in the best of health for centuries by adhering to these type of dietary regimes, albeit unaware they were exercising food law principles, I believe God will still bless anyone who keeps his Laws wether they be Christian or otherwise, This book is primarily all about Health & wellbeing, How to achieve it & how to keep it, this is why the benefits are equally applicable to anyone of any persuasion, Religious, Racial, or otherwise, The reason for writing this book was Threefold.

First,....Many of the books dealing with the Dietary laws of God have been in circulation for many years, & over this long period they do not, with the exception of a few, appear to have had a very profound effect on the health & wellbeing of the man in the street, Twenty First Century citizens in particular appear to have abandoned totally these Laws designed for our physical & mental health, "They are destroyed for lack of knowledge" and many "Because they have rejected knowledge" (Hosea 4-6) David the King & Psalmist of Israel lamented when his fugitive son Abner left the safety of the City of Refuge & was assassinated & said, "Died Abner as a fool dieth" (2 Samuel 3-v27-39) many people (& Christians in particular) are like Abner, they are ill or dying because they have left the safety of Gods word, & rejected the safety of Gods Laws & are indulging in the same dietary practices as the heathen nations of old, is it any wonder they are sick or dying ? Is it any wonder many are not healed?

Settle this in your head. **It is not Gods plan to keep you alive without eating & It is not Gods plan to keep you Well without eating Right,** I feel, having read some of these books & other similar ones, that the principal issues are not defined forcefully enough with the result that the point does not get through to the reader in a positive manner, many of these books pussyfoot around,& do not address the real issue, they are stifled by niceties & literary etiquette, I feel the time has come when a spade has got to be called a spade, & blunt language has got to be used where necessary to ensure the reader is in no doubt as to the serious nature of what is being said or implied.

The Second reason is the need for a fuller understanding of the workings of the Medical & Pharmaceutical establishments & the role they play in our everyday lives. Being a Doctor is not just a job, it's a Vocation & we should be able to trust them with our lives, Alas it is becoming more hazardous to our health to do this & in order to survive in the medical jungle we need to be better informed, preferably from a source that is not biased & is qualified to advise us without fear or favour, **Thirdly** & More personal, it makes me sad to see my numerous friends both Christian & non Christian alike stricken with illnesses that are not only preventable but also curable by adopting. the relatively simple & logical principles of the Creators Food laws, Non Christians could be excused for not knowing about these Divine dietary principles but what is sad is that many Christians do not know about these laws either, & the ones that do know indulge in wilful disobedience virtually every time they eat, & they are highly offended if the subject of healthy food or diet is mentioned in their presence," **Their belly is their God"** (philippians ch.3 -.19) is an apt description of these people. It may not be polite or indeed the thing to do in these days of political correctness to call someone a Glutton, but this is Biblical language & overrides Political correctness & mans ideals, judging from the excess baggage many Christians

(& non Christians) carry around on their bodies in the form of Flab (or "Adipose tissue" if you prefer the medical term), no other word is appropriate (proverbs ch.23:21) if the Bible uses this language to describe Obese & very overweight individuals why should I be any different? But this state of affairs need not be & I will be showing you how to get back on track.(assuming, that is, you were on track in the first place).

How many times have you heard it said that the Devil is making an all out attack on Gods servants in these last days & especially his Ministers, through illness? I, like many others believed this at one time, but I now have reservations, I think it is too convenient to blame the Devil for misfortunes Gods servants may well be the authors of themselves, The Devil is responsible for a lot of things, but there are also a lot of things for which he is **not** responsible,& it is very possible that Gods Ministers & Christians in general have used this as an excuse to avoid taking responsibility for their own actions, it is not enough to say "The devil made me ill," the Devil will take advantage of your weakness or vulnerability if you have an illness but in general terms if you have an illness (apart from an illness caused directly or indirectly by trauma, or environmental factors) more often than not its because you have brought it on yourself through your diet &/or lifestyle, the resultant illness could well be the accumulation of years of unhealthy dietary preferences, either knowingly or unknowingly, **Arthritis, Heart problems, Circulatory problems, Renal problems(Oedema, Fluid retention, Nephritis, Gout, ect.--) Endocrine disorders eg.- (Diabetes types 1&2, Digestive & Kidney diseases) Cancer,** to name but a few, These do not come about overnight, they are caused usually by years of dietary abuse, resulting in an imbalance in the body's metabolism & a lack of vital nutrients which have allowed free radicals (rogue cells) to build up & rampage & erode the vital elements necessary to protect your body from these illnesses, being a Minister of the Gospel does not make you immune from Disease, Your body is the Temple of the Holy Ghost & should be treated as such, if you treat your body like God intended your health problems should be minimal & you should be fit, physically as well as spiritually for the masters use, think on this the next time you feel the Devil is physically, or mentally, persecuting you (which he may well be doing) & make a close scrutiny of your diet & your lifestyle, this is very likely where you will find the answer to your problems.

Yours sincerely,

Tom Pritchard

CHAPTER 1

THE LAWS OF GOD

"MAN WAS DESIGNED FOR ACCOMPLISHMENT, ENGINEERED FOR SUCCESS, & ENDOWED WITH THE SEEDS OF GREATNESS".—Zig Ziglar. (1)

The Universe is governed by a set of laws. The Sun the Moon and the Galaxies did not come into being by chance, nor do they continue to exist or function by chance, they are all subject to Universal laws, the laws of God., the origin of matter & indeed life itself still remains unanswered by the Atheist & the Evolutionist which is basically why Evolution is still referred to as a "Theory" & not a "Fact," The fact that belief in a Divine being & Creator is not just the domain of the ignorant savage or the ordinary, average man is very apparent when we see many prominent & very eminent Scientists & other public luminaries testify of their faith & belief in God, indeed men like Sir Isaac Newton, regarded universally as the greatest Scientist of all time, who gave us the Theory of Gravity & planetary motion, The basis of the laws of Mass, Momentum,& Inertia was established by him, The picture of the Universe reveals Law, Order,& Precision, Newton was once quoted as saying,-- "Hypoththeses non fingo"which in Latin meant he did not deal with mere Suppositions,Other earlier & contemporary scientists who stated their belief in God include men like, Sir Francis Bacon 1561 1626 (Philosophy & reason) Johannes Kepler 1571-1630 mathematician &Astronomer(Developed the Laws of Planetary motion) Galileo Galilei 1564-1642(theory of dynamics) Lord Kelvin 1824-1907(Physicist developed the Second law of Thermodynamics

& the Kelvin Temperature scale) James Clarke Maxwell 1831-1879(Physicist,developed the science of Electromagnetism,) Max Planck 1858-1947(Physicist, developed Quantum theory & Thermodynamics) Albert Einstein 1879-1955(Physicist, Developed Theory of Relativity)A few modern day scientists include---Dr.William Curtis lll (Aeronautical &Nuclear Physics) Dr.Raymond v. Damadian (Pioneer of Magnetic Resonance Imaging) Dr. Robert Herrmann (Professor of mathematics ,U.S. Naval academy) These are just a few of the multitudes of highly educated & prominent scientists, who believed in God & creation.

More recently19th.&20th.Century luminaries like.Benjamin Disraeli,(ProminentBritishPolitician)-QueenVictoria,David Livingstone, Abraham Lincoln, Lord Tonypandy (ex speaker of the House of Lords),-Field marshal Viscount Montgomery of Alamein-& so we could go on, ad infinitum.

Nuclear science & Physics is not confined to the twentieth century ,these are things that were mentioned in the Bible thousands of years ago, but it was not until our modern scientific knowledge increased that we realized the Bible had spoken of these scientific events, our limited scientific knowledge prevented us from interpreting these scientific biblical statements until relatively recent times, Think about some of these statements, Exodus19.v12 -13 "And thou shall set bounds unto the people round about (Mount Sinai) saying, Take heed that ye go not up into the mount or touch the border of it, there shall not a hand touch it ,but he shall surely be **STONED** or **SHOT THROUGH** whether it be beast or man"(this was when Moses was on mount Sinai speaking with God on the peoples behalf) what makes this statement so special is the fact that it uses two words that are confined to Nuclear science EG.**"Stoned"** & **"Shot through"**, These are terms used when someone ,or thing is penetrated with **Radiation,** if the dosage is high enough, it can be fatal, It is believed that mount Sinai was surrounded with high intensity radiation around the perimeter, hence the divine warning, But Nuclear science was not confined to the Old Testament ,it is also mentioned prophetically in the New Testament, speaking of the end times Matthew24.-v29states "Immediately after the tribulation of those days (just prior to the second coming) the sun shall be darkened & the moon shall not give his light & the **Powers of the Heavens shall be shaken",** These words may seem insignificant but they have a special meaning, the Greek rendering of the word **"Powers"** is **DUNAMIS** from which we get our English word **"DYNAMITE"** (the explosive)The Greek word for **Heavens** is **"URANUS"** (or **OURANOS**) & the English derivative of this is **"URANIUM",** This is a classic example of the process of Nuclear fission when Atomic weapons are exploded, **"URANIUM 235"** is the principle element in Nuclear weapons & it is highly unstable, it is composed of 2 Isotopes which are safe enough when kept apart but when they come together by means of an explosive trigger they set off a nuclear reaction, the end result of which is a Nuclear explosion resulting in...total devastation, The Bible writers did not know they were describing Nuclear warfare, but we know this now, Do you still believe the Bible is dull & Uninteresting & Unscientific?.

The Bible is not just scientifically accurate in its language it is also more up to date than tomorrows newspapers.

All Major events of any significance in World history have been Prophesied,& indeed most of these events have already taken place, What, you may ask, has all this got to do with the Food Laws,? Well what I have attempted to do is to show you in some small detail the Scientific Accuracy of the Bible, when the very elite of the worlds intelligentsia can relate to it & see divine intelligence behind nature & creation & understand that everything had a beginning including life itself then we begin to understand why the Bible says "The fool hath said in his heart, "There is no God,"(Psalm 53v.1) The meticulous planning that went into the creation of the Universe also went into the creation of our bodies and the foods that provide the nutrients to maintain & build up our bodies, this is why God gave us a set of guidelines & a list of foods that would be beneficial to us, Our bodies are designed to operate & function within certain limits,(just like the Universe) these limits can be stretched, but only so far, The Food Laws were designed to facilitate the healthy operation & function of our bodies through superior nutrition,

Man is like the food he was designed to eat, he came from the ground originally, just like his food & he returns to the ground when he dies, his life is designed & centred around nature, his body was never designed to assimilate artificial food, artificial food is dead, man was meant to eat living food, like Plants, Herbs, Fruit, Vegetables, Fish, & certain Animals,(notice I said Certain, not All animals) it is these things that keep him healthy.

CHAPTER 2

THE LAW OF CAUSE & EFFECT

The Christian and non-Christian alike is subject to the laws of God. The most fundamental of these is the law of Cause and Effect, e.g.,-**"For every effect there is a cause"** or, a similar law, **"The law of the Harvest"** as it is described in the bible, eg: **"Whatsoever a man soweth that shall he also reap",** If you disregard these laws you will pay the penalty no matter who or what you are., being a Christian will not make you immune from the effects of breaking these laws, There are also other laws which the creator instituted for our health & wellbeing, these are the Dietary, or Food Laws as they are better known. What you put into your body (& when) determines how your body will react and also how you will feel, your body may not react immediately indeed it may not react for hours, days, or even months, or possibly even years, but eventually it will start to exhibit signs & symptoms of what you have been feeding it, if it has been properly nourished your body will reflect this in the way you look, feel, & think, yes, think---if you look, & feel good this affects the way you think, The Immune system releases chemicals called "Cytokines" which stimulate the production of "Serotonin", which in turn regulates mood, so the more healthy your immune system is the better you feel, both Mentally & Physically, so it pays to keep your Immune system in high gear, Antidepressants, who needs them, boost your Immune system instead & get a Serotonin boost, (this is the body's Antidepressant)If on the other hand you feed your body devitalized, lifeless food you will look devitalized & lifeless because your body will reflect it, this in turn will affect your mood, general health & the way you think & usually give rise to numerous ailments which will in turn be easy to get but hard to shift because your immune system will have been starved of vital nutrients for so long it will be ineffective, also it will have been hammered even more by any vaccines you may have had.(see chapter 10)

The food laws are not rocket science, they are common sense, but alas Common sense is not very common, The master Nutritionist, God himself, designed our bodies and knows what is best for us, and he gave us a Maintenance Manual, a set of dietary laws for us to follow in order to maintain perfect health, John the Apostle in The third epistle of John (verse2) states **"Beloved I wish above all things that thou mayest prosper and be in health, even as thy soul prospereth"**, It is Gods will for you to be in good health but you must play your part, you must be obedient to Gods law, if you are obedient and keep these laws to the best of your ability you will enjoy good health all your days, but if you decide you know best and disregard these laws, you will pay the penalty in your body with

Ill health, Pain, Misery and possibly premature death, Christians(& also non Christians) all over the world have, for years been paying the price of disobedience, in many cases because of ignorance of Gods law, Just as ignorance of the laws of the land is no excuse in the eyes of a judge so too ignorance of Gods laws is no excuse in Gods eyes, This ignorance has come about partly because they have never been taught by their spiritual leaders or Shepherd's, in many cases their Shepherd's indulge in the same unhealthy dietary practices as they do,& this is evident when you look at the sheer bulk of many Pastors, Gods Ministers will be judged for the **"Sin of Omission"** if they have failed to instruct the people in these important laws of God without fear or favour, wether it be a popular subject or not.

There is a very popular notion among many Christians that the Mosaic Laws do not apply to us any more, because, as they put it, **"We are not under Law but under grace"** (Romans 6-14-15) does this also apply to the **10 Commandments?** They are Mosaic laws! The fact is, wether you like to believe it or not we are still duty bound by other

Mosaic laws which were given for our Health & welfare not only of the individual but Society in general, these laws are eg :

1 **The Civil Law** (to maintain law, order & justice)

2 **The Criminal law** (to punish the criminal according to the severity of the crime) this included Corporal punishment (flogging or birching) for Antisocial behaviour eg...Mugging, Social disturbance, Persistent offenders, etc. Bullies & Muggers & violent criminals understand Pain &usually learn from it as was demonstrated in the Isle of Man(U.K.Dependency up until 1975.) until the Government went soft on crime,& abolished birching there, up until corporal punishment was abolished on the orders of the British Government, the Isle of Man had the lowest crime rate in the whole of the U.K., after the abolition the crime rate soared, I think it is fair to say that Solomon's instruction to Parents in Proverbs ch.13.v24 "He that spareth the rod hateth his son but he that loveth him chasteneth him betimes(or, when necessary)" could also be equally applied to the Government but the E.U.,s Human Rights

legislation has effectively handcuffed the Law & virtually liberated the criminal. (2)

The Criminal law also included Capital punishment for Murder, which was instituted by God as the ultimate punishment for the ultimate crime, God did not change his mind on this, because," **I am the Lord I change not** "nor did he permit swapping capital punishment for a life sentence (Numbers 35..vI6-33) Did Jesus disagree with this? I think not, after all he was God & he made these laws, when he denounced Jewish justice ,eg.- "An eye for an eye, & a tooth for a tooth"(Matthew 6-38) he was referring to revenge tit for tat style killings & kangaroo courts which the Jews indulged in, he was not denouncing the death penalty, because legalized judicial executions for pre-meditated murder is Biblical & God ordained,& still applies today, just like it did in Bible times, Murder is still Murder, So is the Executioner guilty of murder also since he is the one who sends the criminal into Eternity, Many people including Christians who oppose the Death penalty would say YES, But this is not what the Bible says, According to the Bible, the Executioner is **absolved** because he is doing the will of God according to God's law, read (Numbers 35-v27)"**And the avenger of blood (executioner) kill the slayer, he shall NOT be guilty of blood"**. Do you know the Law better than God? No matter how distasteful the Death penalty may be it is still the Law of God, it was given as a punishment, wether or not it acts as a deterrent is immaterial, you cannot pick & choose which Laws you want & which Laws you don't. The Eighth commandment says "Thou shalt not kill", God regarded life as sacred, & not to be taken lightly which is why he instituted the Death penalty, because Murder in Gods eyes was the ultimate crime & demanded the ultimate penalty. Another crime which was punishable by death was **Homosexuality,** or **Sodomy** as the Bible calls it, Gays or Lesbians were not to be tolerated in any shape or form, where does it say this? Leviticus 20v13 **"If a man also lie with mankind (another man), as he lieth with a woman both of them have committed an abomination, they shall surely be put to death, their blood shall be upon them."** so much for Gay Christians, the Bible knows no such thing. Homosexuality is not in your genes neither is it a freak of nature that cannot be helped, it is sexual deviance, & is classed as sin; there can be no argument unless you wish to argue with God.

3 **The Economic Law**(to ensure a fair & accountable system of Governmental financial management)

4 **The Agricultural law** (to ensure adequate, wholesome, & pesticide free food, grown in healthy mineral rich soil)

5 **The Health law** (to ensure the best health & welfare system ever seen)The old Ceremonial & Temple laws dealing with daily Sacrifices & similar such ordinances were the outdated laws which Paul was referring to when he said **"We are not under law"** It is true we are not under **THESE** laws because the sacrifice of Jesus on the cross done away with the sacrifices offered daily by the high Priest,. Jesus was **"Sacrificed once for all"** but this by no means nullifies the other Laws(outlined above) given originally for the health & social welfare of ancient Israel, & passed down to us for our health & social wellbeing These Laws were not meant to be taken lightly, because they govern every aspect of our life, to keep us

Healthy, Wealthy, & Wise, & be an example to a world that has abandoned God & his ways & has paid the price for doing things **"My Way."**

CHAPTER 3

THE BASICS OF THE FOOD LAWS
(LEVITICUS CHAPTER 11)

ALL SCAVENGERS, BE THEY ANIMALS, BIRDS, SEA CREATURES, OR INSECTS, ARE, ACCORDING TO THE FOOD LAWS, UNCLEAN, & THEREFORE UNFIT FOR HUMAN CONSUMPTION.

Outlined below is a brief summary of some of these.

SHELLFISH....Lobsters...Octopus, Cuttlefish, Starfish, Shrimps, Prawns, Cockles, Mussels, Crabs, Oysters plus All creatures which creep or crawl in the seas or rivers, These are among the most common shellfish found in Fishmongers & Supermarkets, these are primarily "bottom dwellers," They live mostly on the seabed & feed on plankton & dead or contaminated matter which drifts down to the seabed from the surface,

ALL sea scavengers are Unclean, & according to the Food Laws are Unfit for human consumption.

Shellfish & the various types of Shellfish poisoning.

Shellfish are forbidden in the food laws because they are unclean, needless to say they are very popular even among Christians, primarily because little or nothing is known about the potential health hazards of shellfish, very little emphasis is ever put on the consumption of shellfish because it is mostly the eating of meats that gets all the attention, shellfish seem to be of secondary importance, but in terms of relative health the consumption of shellfish is very important primarily because of the high toxicity levels found among some species of sea scavengers The shellfish feed on Plactonic Algae which can be very toxic depending on where the shellfish are harvested, According to the American F.D.A.(food & drug administration) Centre for Food Safety & Applied Nutrition There are 4 principal types of shellfish poisoning,e.g.- **.P.S.P,.D.S.P,.N.S.P. ,A.S.P.**

PSP is short for **Paralytic Shellfish Poisoning** & is generally the most severe, this is a combination of up to 20 toxins, the species usually affected are **MUSSELS, CLAMS, COCCLES & SCALLOPS**, the side effects are generally neurological & include--Tingling in the extremities, Numbness, Drowsiness, Incoherent speech, Respiratory Paralysis which can lead to death in severe cases or in older people or those with a weak immune system, symptoms can occur within 5 minutes to 2 hours, the severity depending on the amount consumed.

D.S.P. is short for **Diarrheic Shellfish Poisoning**. This is usually the mildest form of poisoning & symptoms are usually Diarrhoea, Nausea, and Vomiting some times leading to dehydration especially in older people due to loss of fluids.

N.S.P. or Neurotoxic shellfish poisoning (Polyethers or Brevtoxins),is characterized by Gastro intestinal & Neurological symptoms namely e.g. Diarrhoea, Vomiting, Tingling sensations, Numbness of lips tongue & throat, Muscular aches, Dizziness, Reversal of sensations, e.g. Hot & Cold.

A.S.P. OR **Amnesic** shellfish poisoning, symptoms are e.g. Abdominal pain, Confusion, Memory loss, Disorientation, Seizure, Coma.

Amnesiac poisoning & **Paralytic** poisoning are the two most lethal forms of shellfish poisoning & the severity of the side effects vary with the amount consumed & also the state of health of the individual. Shellfish, although they may be tasty morsels, & some may also be taken for their Aphrodisiac properties this does not reduce their potential to do real damage & play havoc with the bodies systems, so it's yet again a case of Consumer Beware,!!! ….Gods word has warned you,!! You will not see any warnings in the shops.

FISH. All fish that have not got Fins or Scales are unclean, The unclean fish are many & varied ,Shark.. Whale..Eel, Seal, Dolphin, Ray, Turtle, Catfish, Stonefish, Mackerel, Sturgeon (from which comes Caviar) Dogfish.

The fish which are **CLEAN** & fit for human consumption according to the Food laws eg.-Herring,Haddock,Halibut,Hake,Whiting,Cod,Pollock,Smelt,Anchovies…Salmon, Trout, Perch..Etc…

THE ANIMALS DEEMED AS UNCLEAN

ALL CARNIVORES (Meat eaters).. Dogs, Cats, Lions, Tigers, Hyenas...etc.

ALL SCAVENGERS, Hyenas, Lions (sometimes) Pigs (both wild & domestic). All animals that walk on 4 paws.

...Snakes (they are carnivores in the sense that they eat other animals as well as plants or grass) Crocodiles, Alligators.

OTHER ANIMALS DEEMED UNCLEAN.

Rabbits, Hares, Rodents., Lizards, Swans, Ducks, Geese, Cormorant Heron, &. Every Creeping thing that flies & also all creeping things that have more than 4 legs.

Scavenger birds such as, Seagulls, Crows, Ravens, Vultures, Eagles, Condors etc..... These birds & others in this category are unclean by virtue of the fact that they are aerial scavengers & will eat dead animals as well as living ones..

THE CLEAN ANIMALS.

Sheep, Goats, Cows, Ox, Bison, Deer (venison) Game birds Chicken, Turkey, Locust, Grasshopper.

There are obviously more animals that could be included, the list is numerous, suffice to say the Biblical definition is," Every beast that parteth the hoof & cleaveth the cleft into two claws & cheweth the cud among the beasts, that shall you eat".

There are numerous other animals which part the hoof (or, cloven hoof as it is known) but they DO NOT CHEW THE CUD, These are unclean.

There are also various animals that chew the cud but they do not part the hoof, these also are unclean.

The Food Laws do not stop at living creatures they also encompass Fruits & Vegetables & Nuts,& Plants, but there are Edible & Non-Edible plants,& we must know which is which.

This distinction must be made because there are many dangerous Plants which cannot be eaten because they are poisonous, but many of these plants can be used for making medical compounds to treat numerous Ailments (see list in chapter 14)

OTHER FOODS INCLUDED IN THE FOOD LAWS & LISTED AS EDIBLE, EG

...Grapes,Apricots,.Blueberries,Blackberries,Strawberries,OrangesLemons,limes, Pomegranates, Apples, Peaches, Bananas, etc...

SEEDS are usually discarded when the fruits are eaten but the Levitical food law recommendation is that the seeds of all good fruits are nutritionally beneficial & should be consumed also with the fruit.

NUTS are beneficial as well also the kernels of fruits such as Apricots, Plums, Peaches etc... also Natural Pure Honey,(Manuka or similar) as opposed to cheap mass produced Honey which is little more than sugared syrup.

DAIRY products are also good but need to be monitored for their level of purity & just how free they are of artificial contaminants.

COWS MILK would normally be beneficial but not only is it liable to be contaminated with the numerous drugs & steroids the poor old cow is injected with during its life but also the Pasteurization process eliminates a lot of the nutrients that would normally be in it. If milk is desired or needed, the best by far is GOATS

MILK, the taste is not that much different & it is a heck of a lot purer, as well as more nutritious, Most good Supermarkets stock it, although it is fair to say there is not exactly a mad rush for it, although strictly speaking, there should be if you wish to improve your health prospects, its really a simple matter of adapting to change,...

EGGS are good, but in moderation & not for breakfast, unless you rise at 11 am or so.

CHEESE is also good but depending on the type of cheese & how it is processed it can be dangerous to those with High Cholesterol because some cheeses are very high in their fat content, again the old Goats cheese is as good as any, probably not as tasty, nor as easy to find except in large Supermarkets.

CHAPTER 4

THE PURPOSE OF THE FOOD LAWS

The purpose of the food laws was, and indeed

still is, to put into operation a dietary regime on a national level as well as an individual level that would be highly beneficial, not only to the individual, but the nation as a whole. This regime would ensure the greatest healthcare system the world had ever seen because it would virtually eliminate disease through superior nutrition and hygiene without the use of drugs or unnatural medicines. The purpose of the food laws was also to demonstrate to the world (or in bible times, the non-Israelite nations) the wisdom of god through his superior system of healthcare and the ability of his people to live healthy and long lives through obedience to his food laws.

Our bodies were originally designed to last forever, the bodies we now have are basically the same, except, their physiology has been altered so that regeneration of our worn out cells ceases to take place after a certain number of years. In bible times, just after Adam, and up to the time of the flood, this regeneration process ceased around 800 years (the average lifespan then was around 500 - 800 years(with a few exceptions such as Noah and Methuselah) after the flood this came down to

200 - 400 years until, by the time of Sodom and Gomorrah this long lifespan had dwindled to 70 – 80 years with some exceptions of 100 – 120 years. The purpose of the food laws was, and still is, to educate the people to eat only foods that would be beneficial to maintain the bodies regeneration & healing process and assist the proper functioning of all the bodies systems, thus enabling us to live long & healthy lives as our original forefathers did.

If we adhere to Gods dietary principles we should not require modern medicine with its host of side effects, our bodies were not designed to tolerate drugs because they are alien to the bodies systems, modern science has eventually realized this & attempted to overcome the bodies resistance by using herbal based drugs, some of which are very useful ,like ,eg.-

Digitalis (heart problems)

Anabasis sphylla (skeletal muscle relaxant)-**BerberisVulgaris**(dysentery)-

BetulaAlba(anticancerous)

Erythroxylum coca (local anaesthetic) All these are good & have been used for centuries in their raw natural state by many cultures but natural cures cannot be patented, so the Pharmaceutical companies make synthetic copies of these herbal drugs & make a fortune, unfortunately these copies are not exact &often the side effects are numerous,& sometimes disastrous.

CHAPTER 5

THE RELEVANCE OF THE FOOD LAWS

Ever since Peter the apostle saw the vision of the clean & unclean beasts & birds & creepy crawlies being let down in the sheet, Christians have assumed that this was a licence from God to disregard the food laws & eat anything that had legs or wings wether clean or unclean, that took our fancy & God would protect us from any ill effects we suffered as a result of eating them (Acts ch.10.-10-16) This is not only a fantasy, but also a gross misinterpretation of the whole passage, VERSE 28 gives the true meaning of this vision

"And he (Peter) said unto them Ye know how that it is an unlawful thing for a man that is a Jew to keep company of someone of another nation, but God hath shown me that I should not call any **Man** common or unclean".

The Gentiles were regarded as unclean(Like the unclean beasts & birds in the vision),but God was telling Peter they were no longer Unclean,& the gospel was for them also, & not just the Jews, The vision had nothing at all to do with the food laws or the consumption of animals wither clean or unclean, So what creatures were unclean then are still unclean now, the gospel or the New testament dispensation has not made unclean animals or birds or sea creatures any cleaner or less toxic They are still **Unclean** & still a threat to our health.

The food laws have never had more relevance than in the twenty first century because of the massive increase in fast foods and the huge increase in the consumption of meats and animals which do not conform to the dietary laws of God, and are deemed by God to be unfit for human consumption. The greed for money has led men to use virtually every part of every animal, disguised and packaged and promoted in the supermarkets as good foods. The Israelites of old were surrounded by nations who were plagued by disease because of their indiscriminate pagan diets which allowed them to eat virtually anything they liked, whether clean or unclean. Pigs and all manner of other scavenger animals and birds were included in their diet and they paid the price in disease and premature death, Egypt was a classic example of this, they were plagued by every major disease, the very same diseases the West is plagued with now, the Egyptians had them 3000 years ago, e.g. **Arthritis, Cancer, Heart disease, Diabetes, Arterio Sclerosis, Endocrine disorders** e.g. **Thyroid, Renal and Pancreatic disorders,** you name it & they had it, God knew all these diseases were diet related and promised the Israelites **"If thou will diligently harken to the voice of the lord thy god and will do that which is right in his sight, and will give ear to his commandments and keep all of his statutes I will put none of these diseases upon thee which I have brought upon the Egyptians, for I am the lord that healeth thee"** (Exodus 15:26). The Israelites remained free of disease while they kept the food laws, In these days of rampant diseases are these laws not relevant to us? The cost to the health service and the country in general from sickness and disease is phenomenal, I don't need to tell you about the acute shortage of hospital beds due to the increasing number of people with medical maladies of one sort or another, all this translates into money which the government has to recoup through taxes paid by the people, Think of the equally phenomenal scenario if the people were encouraged to practice food law principles and eat only wholesome meats and foods according to Bible principles, the savings to the health service through the vast reduction of patients requiring medical attention would be unbelievable, not to mention the savings for the government exchequer in unnecessary drugs and treatments which rake in billions of pounds annually for the Pharmaceutical industry..Healthcare costs will rise as long as Drug demand & drug prices continue to rise, Drug companies will continue to make Billions of Pounds/ Dollars in profits, much of it at the Tax payers expense.

The solution is to redirect Health Service spending

to create programmes to build up the Peoples health & improve care & help them to help themselves to be more productive & less dependant on Doctors & drugs.

The extra productivity would eventually create more wealth & make healthcare for those who require it a lot cheaper.

The key is to concentrate on Health & wellness & the **Prevention** of disease, rather than treating it after the fact, the vast majority of modern medicines are designed to treat the symptoms, not the actual root cause, these Drugs are not designed to cure ailments but rather to alleviate the symptoms, that is not to say modern medicine could not come up with a cure for many of the worlds ills, they probably could but that would kill their Cash Cow, the good old Repeat proscription. It's a vicious circle, a real dog.

Building up your Immune system is probably one of the best, if indeed not The best method of protection & prevention of Disease in your body, Remember," Disease cannot thrive in the presence of a healthy Immune system",(**not even hereditary ones**) & Raw Fruit (not canned, canned fruit is crammed full of sugars or other types of sweeteners) & Vegetables are the key ingredients in building up this system, not drugs.

In the 1930s a Dentist, Dr.Weston Price undertook a comprehensive study of remote tribal peoples who had not been touched by Western civilization or culture to determine their physical health & lifestyle, he conducted this study on 14 different cultures ranging from Eskimos, Swiss, Polynesian, to African, Pakistani ect---He found an amazingly high standard of health among these people, most had perfect teeth & cavity free even into old age, also they were virtually disease free & had no record or history of cancer or Heart disease also most lived well into old age & still retained a good standard of fitness. The reason or the common denominator for the incredible health of all these people was their lifestyle & their diet which consisted primarily of raw fruits & vegetables, also fish & a variety of nuts, meat was not a regular part of their diet,(the Hunzas of Pakistan consume large amounts of bitter Aipricot seeds which are very high in vitamin B17, they swear by this diet & have been relatively disease free for centuries) Dr. Price wrote a book on his findings which is still a standard textbook on Nutrition, the book is…"Nutrition & Physical Degeneration" by Dr.Weston Price B.D.S. Ernst T.Krebs jnr. The man who pioneered Metabolic therapy 70 odd years ago also conducted an identical survey of remote tribes & got identical results to Dr. Price, The Hunza was one of the tribes he worked closely with.

While on the subject of Medicine & Hospitals some statistics may be of interest to you, & also a little bit of Greek,.

Iatros=Physician

Genic=Disease ,. **Iatrogenic** Disease or death, that is,..Disease or death caused by Doctors or any medical intervention involving drugs, or treatment performed by any Health Professional. On 30/07/2000 Professor Dr. Barbara Starfield MD.MPH of the Johns Hopkins school of Hygiene & Public Health said in the "Journal of American Medicine" that **"Iatrogenic Medicine was the third largest cause of death in the U.S. next to Heart Disease & Cancer,"**. Killing at least 250,000 people a year. (3)

In 2000 in the U.S.A. A Presidential task force labelled "Medical errors" as a national problem of "epidemic proportions", accounting for **60,000-100,000** deaths in hospital & overall a conservative average of **240,000** deaths from Medical interventions of one sort or another, The Centre for Disease control &Prevention estimate **2,000,000** people annually contract infections while hospitalized & **90,000** die from these infections ,more than 70% of hospital acquired infections are resistant to at least one of the commonly proscribed antibiotics due to over proscribing by physicians & these are only some of the conservative figures for the United States & it's a similar picture for the U.K.& Europe, WHAT A DISASTER! This is the price we pay for deviating from the Biblical food & hygiene principles, ,remember the old law of Cause & Effect! "For every effect there is a cause",apart from Trauma the cause is almost always of dietary origin ,remember the law of Cause & Effect, & eat accordingly & you will stay healthy & quite possibly live to old age, and if you are able to stay out of Hospitals you definitely have a head start for living to Old Age.

CHAPTER 6

THE RELEVANCE OF THE FOOD LAWS TO INDUSTRY

We all know that sickness takes a heavy toll on industry through lost time. One of the biggest problems of any employer, especially the smaller ones, is budgeting for health related absenteeism. Medical analysts believe much of this sickness is Psychosomatic, or in layman's terms, the illness is genuine but the cause is rooted in the mind, frequently these causes are Boredom, Stress and job Discontentment, poor quality, fast food lunches don't help either. Very frequent causes of sickness are stomach and back problems, nine times out of ten the stomach problems are due to intestinal bugs (infections), & to a lesser degree, ulcers, all of these are due to poor diet, poor nutrition and in many cases binging the night before either on fast foods or alcohol or both. Infected meats (especially pork, bacon and ham & other cooked meats) are a primary source of infection & in some cases can be particularly lethal, all this has a detrimental effect not only on the individual, who could lose not only his job, but also his house if he cannot keep up his mortgage repayments (many thousands of houses are repossessed annually because of this as of September 2007 the annual repossession number was 14,000),this is also a serious blow to industry generally, in reduced production, lost contracts, reduced profits,& if this state of affairs continues, layoffs, this in turn affects other smaller subsidiaries, or suppliers, which were dependant on the larger company for orders,.& all this (apart from injury) because of sickness which might well have been prevented with proper diet & eating habits, Also if the company is forced to close because of reduced financial income & mounting financial overheads this contributes to a reduction in the Governments GNP.-the "Gross National Product."

Napoleon Bonaparte once said we were a nation of "Small Shopkeepers"& he was right, the multitude of small businesses in the U.K.demonstrates the independent entrepreneurial spirit of independence of our people as well as many foreign peoples who have settled here, the success of these businesses depends on the workforce & for the business to succeed the workforce needs to be reliable, This is why Health is a major factor in keeping the wheels of industry turning, so stay healthy & make Great Britain great again.

CHAPTER 7

THE RELEVANCE OF THE FOOD LAWS TO THE INDIVIDUAL

U.K. citizens are fortunate in that the National Health Service provides free medical services and hospitalization, also the U.K. has reciprocal agreements with other countries. Unfortunately this is not the case in many other countries where medical services must be paid for by the individual and are very expensive, so the less medical attention you need the better, since most common ailments and diseases stem from poor nutrition or poor sanitation it is logical for the individual to make a radical change in his diet and lifestyle & adopt a proven healthy and nutritious range of foods, unfortunately these are not always easy to find, primarily because much of our food is contaminated with toxic pesticides (80% of free fruit for schools was found to be contaminated with pesticide residue) (4) & even the ground they grow in is contaminated with toxic fertilizers designed to force the land to yield its food more quickly,& kill weeds at the same time, all the natural chemical elements & minerals found in good land & ultimately passed on in the food is destroyed because of the chemicals forced into the soil to speed up production & growth, the land is worked so hard it eventually dies, land is like people, it needs a rest to recuperate, in Bible times the land was left to rest one year in every seven & the farmer rested all his fields in rotation so that all his fields were rested one year in every seven, the fertilizers were also natural ensuring the best feeding for the land & ultimately the best quality foods & disease & ailment free people, All this is a thing of the past & we are paying for the error of our ways & the greed of our Politicians, our farmers have to produce more for less, but alas in this case you cannot have Quality & Quantity & the result is devitalized substandard food with barely enough nutrition to sustain a bird let alone a person, the farmer is forced to adopt these measures to maintain a viable living standard, Once again we are seeing that men certainly do not know better than God even though evidently they think they do. G.M.(Genetically Modified) foods are another example of man thinking he can improve on Gods creation by forcing chemicals into the ground to produce crops that supposedly are superior in Nutritional content & have a longer shelf life, all this sounds fine except for the fact that many of the chemicals used in the seeds & fertilizer are highly toxic & also destroy other natural (non G.M.) crops in neighbouring fields when the wind blows the G.M.seed pollen across the fields, But it does not stop there, many cases of local communities being affected & manifesting many symptoms of toxic poisoning have been reported, this has been the case especially in the Philippines & other Far East countries where regulations are not so strict, And who manufactures this toxic food? Surprise surprise, **The Pharmaceutical manufacturers**

The logic is simple, if they cant sell it to you one way they will sell it to you another way.

Do you remember the "Mad Cow Disease" **(B.S.E.)** epidemic not so long ago,(1984) when multitudes of cows, healthy or otherwise were slaughtered, Scientists were agreed it was a Viral infection that caused the disease, but they did not know where it originated or how the cows got it, so they slaughtered them all, or most of them, just to be on the safe side.

It is interesting to note that out of all the European countries Switzerland & the U.K. were the only 2 countries to be plagued with **B.S.E.**Its also interesting to note that these were the only 2 countries insisting on the use of the Organophosphate pesticide **Phosmet** A blend of Organophosphates & the base of the drug **Thalidomide**,(do you remember the huge controversy surrounding Thalidomide in the 60s?) I.C.I.manufactured **Phosmet** ,Excessive use of this almost certainly caused the damage, The pesticide is massaged into the skin of the cow to kill Warble flies, it penetrates deep into the flesh & muscle, these Organophosphate toxins affected the animals

Nervous system crossing body barriers & binding with crucial nerve enzymes, disrupting pathways of the C.N.S.(central nervous system) also the Peripheral & Autonomic nervous systems.

One particular farmer, **Mark Purdey** refused to use this stuff on his cattle & significantly none of them got B.S.E. When Purdey refused to use this poison on his animals **M.A.F.F.**(Ministry of Agriculture, Forestry & Fisheries) took him to court to force him to use it but the case was thrown out, the Judge ruled the Government could not force him to use it because the chemical was neither a vaccine nor a serum ,but this was not the end, It is interesting to note that when MR.Purdey tried to work with Government agencies to determine if Phosmet was linked to B.S.E. strange things began to happen, in addition to being shot at & his house burning down, Mr. Purdeys Lawyers & a Vet he was working with all had serious car crashes , two of them fatal, one lawyer & the Vet were killed, the surviving lawyer said he was deliberately run off the road.

After publication of an article in "The Independent" in 1993 Mr. Purdeys phone lines were cut, preventing him from receiving follow up media calls. It seems Toxic chemical research is a dangerous business especially when the manufacturers are annoyed.

Ultimately we, the consumers pay the price, But we don't necessarily have to if we look closely at what we buy & where, it is still possible to find good quality foods, its just a question of shopping around & looking for foods that are nutritionally beneficial & not just tasty or appetizing, The cost of being healthy is a lot less than the cost of being sick, There is so much lethal unclean food (unclean by food law standards, that is) to choose from, every supermarket is virtually a suicides paradise, its men's ideas that have changed, I would call this convenient unbelief,. pure & simple, they are as guilty as the Lords own Disciples when they refused to believe Jesus had risen from the dead , the disciples knew that since he was crucified on Wednesday (not Good Friday as is commonly believed)& was interred in the tomb just before sunset (6pm) he would rise again 72 hours later, I would assume you count 3 days & 3 nights as 72 hours as I do, but Mary Magdalene went to the tomb on Sunday morning with spices to anoint Jesus body fully expecting to find him still in the tomb & when the Angels told her he had risen she was surprised ,even when she saw Jesus in the garden her brain refused to let her believe it was him ,& when she eventually got over the shock & told the disciples she had seen the Lord, they, the Lords own disciples, would not believe her, this would explain why all the disciples disappeared at the crucifixion(except John) they never believed Jesus when he told them he would rise again in 3 days, Even the sisters of Lazarus did not believe Jesus could or would raise Lazarus up there & then & this was why Jesus wept, he was weeping because these, his close friends, did not believe him, not because Lazarus was dead.(he already knew this 4 days previously).

This is like so many believers (or should I say unbelievers) who find it convenient to disregard or simply refuse to believe in the relevance or validity of the Levitical food laws for today, its not convenient for them, the effort involved in being obedient is too much for them, it requires too much effort to sacrifice the unclean foods they love so much.

CHAPTER 8

THE CHRISTIAN & HEALING

This is not an easy subject to comment on because there are so many different aspects & opinions on the subject of healing that it would require a book to do it justice ,suffice to say it is not as straightforward as some Bible expositors, Faith healers & T.V.Evangelists would lead us to believe, It is my opinion that "Jesus Christ is the same yesterday ,today , & forever"(Hebrews 13-8) & he still works miracles & healings today just as he did 2000 years ago ,many healings are unconditional, especially those performed through Missionaries to demonstrate Gods power & love to peoples who have never heard of Jesus ,& sometimes require a sign that he is the God of Gods.(5)

Sometimes God also elects to heal believers unconditionally either through their faith or the faith of the Elders (James 5-14) but there are also many cases when Believers are not healed & the Lord does not always give a reason why. There are also times when God permits sickness to afflict believers to teach them a lesson, especially when the sickness is due to disobedience of Gods food laws, assuming of course we are aware of the food laws & the fact that we are breaking them, if a believer is not aware of the food laws or the fact that they are breaking them their spiritual leaders should enquire of them what their dietary food preferences are & like a Physician instruct them in the laws of God & how they can regain good health (assuming this is the cause, which it generally is), thus preparing the way for the body to heal itself, although having said that it is fair to assume that many Pastors or Elders if you suggested this would probably ask you, "Do you think I am a Doctor"? & the answer is **YES** Pastors & Elders are supposed to be Spiritual Doctors & the Bible is their Spiritual equivalent of **"Greys Anatomy"**.(the Doctors Bible) Elders & Pastors are expected to be Councillors, Instructors, Teachers, Leaders by example, This is what the office calls for & this is the criteria God expects of those who occupy these offices & they should know what is required of them, if they do not fulfil the criteria they should either rectify the situation by study or be true to themselves & to God & vacate the office, Many of Gods people are ill through ignorance, ignorance that could quite easily be rectified with quality counselling, counselling that should come from informed Elders & Pastors.(unfortunately in many churches this counselling is not very evident)

EXODUS.15.26 "I AM THE LORD THAT HEALETH THEE", you would almost think this is the whole verse, so many preachers quote this verse before they call for a healing line & when some people go away the same as they came they begin to wonder, Why am I not healed? The preacher does not always know why(unless God specifically tells him) & this just adds to the confusion because the way the preacher was preaching they were virtually guaranteed to be healed Many preachers or faith healers if you wish to call them that, very rarely quote the whole verse, which gives the conditions for healing ,this is it **"IF THOU WILT DILIGENTLY HARKEN TO THE VOICE OF THE LORD THY GOD**

& WILL DO THAT WHICH IS RIGHT IN HIS SIGHT& WILL GIVE EAR TO HIS COMMANDMENTS & KEEP ALL HIS STATUTES, I WILL PUT NONE OF THESE DISEASES UPON THEE WHICH I HAVE BROUGHT UPON(or allowed to come upon) THE EGYPTIANS......FOR I AM THE LORD THAT HEALETH THEE" ,as you can see there are certain conditions attached to this verse ,its not always as straightforward as some make out, its not always a case of "Believe it & receive It", there are as always some exceptions when God deems to heal someone without pre conditions, but this is the exception rather than the rule & God has his own reasons for these exceptions,. The statutes & commandments mentioned here are the laws laid down for our health & wellbeing, we cannot expect to flout the very laws which were designed to keep us healthy & not reap the consequences of our disobedience.

Once again it's the law of the harvest," whatsoever a man soweth that shall he also reap", God does not often override the laws of nature & if you eat unclean foods or meats you will reap a harvest of sickness & disease & possibly death, God will **NOT** make an exception in your case, he will try to educate you so that you will learn from your mistakes, but as always its better if you learn from the mistakes of others rather than your own, it will not be so painful.

One would think that by now there would be enough examples of disobedience among Christians to make us resolve to be the most conscientious food law adherents on the planet, sadly this is just not the case, the serpent has beguiled us yet again & told us," God understands your weaknesses, a bit of a change is in order now & again, a bit of Pork, or some nice Bacon or Cooked Ham for a start or maybe some nice Crab or Duck, or even the aphrodisiac Cockles & Muscles all unclean & deemed by God unfit for human consumption, Do you know better than God?.

When did you last read the book of LEVITICUS,(Chapter 11) This is where God speaks to you about your health & how to be free of disease & stay free, it is worth more than all the medical text books or so called Good health guides because the author is the designer & creator of our bodies, the mighty God himself, if he says something is unfit for our Consumption, then it is unfit, Period!! To question God's law is detrimental to our health, we should know this by now, but alas we do not seem to have got the message yet. Stop trying to be wiser than God; it could be a painful or even fatal experience.

CHAPTER 9

BODY SYSTEMS

Our bodies are miracles of Divine engineering, designed to be independent & very resilient, It is a multi-role, multi-system powerhouse complete with backup. These systems are able to cope with a certain amount of stress, but to be able to do this it requires fuel to burn & nutrients to sustain & repair itself, given the proper foods it can do amazing things, It can heal itself, It can grow new tissue & new cells, It can even defend itself against invaders, The bodies Immune system is unique, it can detect & identify foreign bodies,(or substances) which are harmful to us & put into operation a series of defensive measures designed to protect our vital organs & retain the bodies integrity, It does not require vaccines to tell it wether a substance is alien to it or not, or wether a substance is harmful to our systems or not, our immune system is designed to detect & destroy anything that is not compatible with the wellbeing of our bodies, the Immune system is a complex of organs, highly specialized cells & even a circulatory system of its own separate from blood vessels ,This is known as the lymphatic system, lymph nodes are dotted all over the body & provide meeting grounds for immune system cells that defend against invaders, there are 2 major types of Immune system cells, the **B** cells & the **T** cells, The B cells produce cells that are basic templates for other cells that target specific antigens, While the **T** cells are more specialized, these regulate & orchestrate the response of an elaborate system of different types of cells such as helper, or **CD4** positive T cells(**CD4+**) there are also other T cells which patrol the blood &

lymph systems monitoring &guarding against foreign bodies T cells also coordinate the overall immune response, the complexity of the immune system is staggering to say the least, it can even tell if a threat to the body is of major or minor proportions, what type of bug or virus it is & order different types of cells to deal with it accordingly, its sensory organs are able to determine the size & nature of the threat &,the response is measured according to that threat, it is not only able to produce a matching antibody for every one of the millions of different infective agents, but is also able to remember the appropriate antibodies for different diseases & produce these same antibodies for the same diseases & infections decades later, What an amazing system this is, boosted & fuelled by vitamins & minerals drawn from various plants, vegetables & fruits, **it does not need help from drugs or vaccines to improve or boost its performance,** it outclasses anything modern medicine has to offer, all it needs is good quality food to maintain its integrity & boost its effectiveness.

Unfortunately this amazing miracle of creation

is often compromised & its effectiveness greatly reduced by the consumption of food which is not compatible with the Body's wellbeing, all these serve only to contaminate the body & starve the immune system, leaving the body defenceless,& vulnerable to every bug & virus that is going around, this is why one of the primary causes of death in Cancer & Aids patients is Heart failure precipitated by repeated Chest& Respiratory tract infections due to their Immune system being shot to pieces by chemotherapy drugs,Dr.Douglas Brodie M.D.(Alternative Cancer therapist) writing in Burton Goldberg,s"**Alternative Medicine definitive guide to Cancer**" in 1997 said "**Each one of us produces several hundred thousand cancer cells every day,whether we develop cancer or not depends upon the ability of our Immune system to destroy these cancer cells, That's because CANCER THRIVES IN THE PRESENCE OF A DEFICIENT IMMUNE SYSTEM**",(6) Incidentally your TONSILS are also part of your immune system, & are there to protect you, when they become inflamed this is a sign of infection when it happens often Doctors are prone to recommending Tonsillectomies to cure the problem (this is the removal of the tonsils by surgery) this is curing the symptoms rather than the root cause which is usually dietary in its nature (It is not at all unusual for Doctors not to know this) Infections are caused by foreign bodies (or "bugs" as they are commonly known) entering our bodies either by trauma or more commonly by infected food (usually contaminated meats), The Tonsils, being part of the Immune system are there to fight the infection & are a part of the bodies defence mechanism, they are not meant to be cut out, if someone is having persistent Tonsillitis this is a sign the person has a dietary deficiency & is consuming contaminated food (meat in particular is usually the prime suspect, being the commonest source of infection) or food that is low in essential nutrients such as fast foods, junk foods & fizzy drinks (usually containing Aspartame as a sweetener, see article on Aspartame) A poor diet reduces the immune systems effectiveness & allows bacteria to multiply & cause havoc,(hence the inflammation) this aspect should be examined closely Tonsillitis has been cured very often by a close scrutiny & regulation of the diet,. Primarily fruit & veg. & a reduction in meat intake, Why is

Common sense so uncommon?

Another alternative consideration is pure **"Manuka Honey"**(Bees get their pollen from the flowers of the Manuka bush) with a U.M.F.factor of at least 10 or above ,the higher the better, it is totally antibacterial & kills all manner of infections (even M.R.S.A.) twice as fast & effective as any thing on the market, its expensive but worth it its also very effective in preventing infections because bugs cannot live in its presence, even when spread on open wounds with a spatula or knife & dressed they also heal far faster than any conventional cream or dressing & since M.R.S.A. is very commonly contracted via open wounds or cuts especially post operatively when surgical wounds are being dressed, or redressed Manuka spread on the wound prior to redressing will help eliminate the possibility of M.r.s.a. infection via this route & help to eliminate this particular bug & also any others(see details & history on internet under Manuka honey,medical uses) As of August 7th.2007 the F.D.A. has approved Manuka honey for medicinal uses & wound dressings, this is the first time it has been approved officially by the

U.S. government, also see the article in the "Daily Mail" 08/07/06 under "Cancer doctors turn to the honey that can heal" Buckwheat Honey is another healer & has very similar properties to Manuka honey.

.ps. It may be of interest to know that any condition or illness with "ITIS" on the end of the name denotes Inflammation which in turn would suggest an infection (although this is not always the case), eg,--Arthr**itis**,-Appendic**itis**, -Tonsill**itis**-- Cyst**itis**, Nephr**itis,** ect.--.,

---It may also be of interest to know that an Oxygen rich body is a healthy body, Disease cannot exist in an oxygen rich body, & the way to keep your body oxygen rich & disease free is through superior nutrition only found in good quality foods, & supplements if necessary, Pathogenic Viruses will not grow where the conditions do not allow it.

CHAPTER 10

VACCINES

The Immune system is also under attack from the least likely source, Vaccines, these are the thing most people have usually depended on to immunize them against infections, given the faith most people put in vaccines it is understandable they will be shocked to learn that this is the last thing they need to immunize them against the numerous bugs going around, Vaccines are "Immunosuppressants",(they suppress the immune system) they are not the magic bullet most people think they are, indeed they compromise the body's Immune system by bypassing the Secretory antibodies within the Respiratory tract mucosa, they bypass this route by being injected into the bloodstream, this leads to a corruption of the Immune system itself & as a result pathogenic Viruses or Bacteria cannot be eliminated by the immune system &

they remain in the body & mutate as the individual is exposed to ever more antigens & toxins, Also the body is further contaminated with Foreign Tissue DNA/RNA found in many vaccines via Graft vs. Host phenomena,(7) The Vaccine Injury Act was passed in the U.S.A.in 1986, since then numerous successful lawsuits totalling billions of dollars were brought against the Government & the Pharmaceutical companies for damage caused by so called "Safe" vaccines, **3,482** claims for compensation totalling **$1.4 Billion** has been paid by Vaccine manufacturers up to Feb.2002, So many claims were being made that a deal was passed in Congress (Dec.2005) granting Pharmaceutical companies immunity from lawsuits, If these vaccines are **"SAFE "**as we are told why are there so many lawsuits for damages? (and these are only the successful lawsuits) On average 11,000 Vaccine injuries are reported each year,& as little as 1% of doctors report any Vaccine related injuries even though by law they are obliged to do so.(8)

In the U.K.£**3.5 Million** has been paid out in Vaccine injury claims between1997, & 2005 In Northern Ireland (Ulster). **£2,000,000** has been paid out to 25 families for children injured by vaccines between 1979-2006 & many believe this is only the tip of the iceberg, because the vaccine injury payment criteria are so deliberately stringent most never qualify for payments even though the claims are genuine. Quite a few of these vaccines have Mercury compounds such as **Thimerosal**,& other similar Neurotoxins the side effects of which can vary & also be quite dangerous, in some cases even fatal, causing damage to the Immune -Sensory-& Neurological systems as well as Motor(movement coordination) & behavioural damage.

The **MMR** vaccine has long courted Controversy, it is thought to be linked to Autism & bowel problems in some types of susceptible children, The Daily Mail of 18/06/06 ran the story of the identical deaths of two 17 month old healthy babies following their vaccination with the MMR jab, the parents were so disgusted with the defiant attitude of the medical authorities they arranged for a piece of brain tissue from each baby to be taken & sent privately to a medical university lab. in America in an effort to verify their suspicions, At the moment as I write this (June 07) a major legal battle is due to take place soon in the supreme court over compensation payments for brain damaged children damaged by the MMR Vaccine, if the court rules in favour of the parents it will open the floodgates for many more such lawsuits & set a precedent making it much easier to claim against the Pharmaceutical giants for damages they knew about but kept quiet about, it is more than obvious the medical profession & the Pharmaceutical companies will go to any lengths to protect their sacred cow even our own Prime Minister refused to state categorically if his own son was immunized with the MMR vaccine, have the Blair's looked up the more accurate insider info on MMR not given to the public? the **SUNDAY OBSERVER 27/08/2000** revealed that the UK government attempted to cover up the deaths of a number of children as a result of the MMR vaccine, but still Governments refuse to do a proper scientific study to see if there is a definite link or not , they say it would cost too much to do a proper scientific study, but the Blair's are not on their own, former U.S. President Bill Clinton on an official visit to the Middle East refused the Anthrax jab, this vaccine is now believed to be at the root of the strange debilitating illness which has virtually immobilized many Gulf war veterans & left many ex-servicemen & women with permanent disability, Already the relatively new 5 in 1 vaccine designed for very young children is giving rise for concern over the side effects many children have had with it so far, & this is only the start.

The latest Vaccine assault on the U.S. population is **"Gardasil"**. Merck pharmaceuticals have developed this for Girls up to the 6th. Grade to immunize them against the sexually transmitted disease H.P.V. which can develop into Cervical Cancer, So far 82cases of serious side effects have been reported since June 2006, & a report in the BMJ (British Medical Journal) on June 9th.2007. said 1,637 cases of adverse side effects had been reported & 3 young girls had died shortly afterwards, The Governor of Texas has tried to persuade the Government to make it mandatory, not optional by 2008 & Merck has lobbied in 18 other States for similar legislation.

As of August 2007 the latest update is that 5 girls have died, 31 have had life threatening side effects, 1385 have had to attend Hospital Casualty departments, 51 have been disabled,& up to July 2007 451 have not recovered as yet from the side effects, The truth of the matter is that H.P.V.is quite easily cured with adequate Sunlight & vitamin D also Selenium & Zinc, experts say that in most cases the condition clears up on its own, also the negative response from parents over the numerous side effects of Gardasil could see this Vaccine off the market,(a course of 3 injections costs $900) A similar vaccine for boys is in the pipeline, We are expected to take chances with vaccines & doctors continue to tell us they are safe, millions of pounds & dollars are spent publicising & pushing them, a proper study would hold up production & cost millions & possibly billions of dollars or pounds in lost profits (and very probably prove the ineffectiveness of the Vaccines) American children are among the most vaccinated in the world, receiving up to **20+** vaccinations within the first 2 years of life & all this in theory is Mandatory, not Optional, at least that is what the Government bodies would like you to believe but in fact there is nothing in Federal Law that makes Vaccination for anyone regardless of age Mandatory, there are Waivers & Clauses both on Religious or Medical grounds by which you can "Opt Out" Check it out with your own State laws, The latest news is that Merck could be going out of business due to the thousands of lawsuits for damages over the painkiller VIOXX.(It is estimated 60,000 have died from this drug since its introduction) (9)

What a disaster, this is not Science, this is Medical & corporate greed & corruption on a vast scale, man has not yet learned that he cannot improve on Gods creation, vaccines are just another source of wealth creation (Doctors & Vets. alike make a hansom profit from vaccines) why do you think the headlines are full of articles about Flu. Pandemics & all manner of other foreign bugs & viruses, which never seem to amount to anything? Its scare tactics, Media Manipulation orchestrated & paid for by those with most to gain, the Pharmaceutical giants & the Medical establishment, backed by the Politicians, to induce the populace both here & abroad to buy the vaccines, this is high pressure sales, with high stakes.

An offer of $75,000 has been made for any Doctor or Pharmaceutical C.E.O.who will publicly drink a mixture of standard vaccine additives, the

additives would be the same as those contained in vaccines recommended for a 6 year old child according to U.S.Centres for disease control & prevention guidelines & the dose would be body weight calibrated., It would include but not be limited to the following Vaccine additives
1..Thimerosal(a Mercury derivative)
2..Ethylene Glycol(antifreeze)
3..Phenol(a disinfectant dye)
4..Aluminum.
5..Benzethonium choloride(disinfectant)
6..Formaldehyde(disinfectant & preservative, used in embalming)

If this offer has not been claimed by August 1st. 2007 the offer will rise to $90,000 & will increase at the rate of $5,000 a month until someone dares to claim it, the man offering the challenge is Jock Doubleday, Director of the California non profit corporation "Natural Woman Natural Man," Not surprisingly this offer has been on the table since 2001 but no one has been willing to take their chances with this chemical cocktail, except for the children who innocently go for routine vaccinations, with the average loans for Medical

students running at well in excess of $100,000 you would think some enterprising Med. Student or Doctor would chance their luck, but then 6 year old children & their Mothers don't ask as many questions as Doctors, nor do they know the risks involved, which is most likely why this generous offer has never been claimed by a Doctor or CEO
In addition to the Viral & Bacterial contaminants that are part of vaccines the following is a list of common Vaccine fillers
Aluminium hydroxide.
Aluminium phosphate.
Aluminium sulphate.
Amphotericin B.
Animal tissues.- Pig blood, Horse blood, Rabbit brain, Dog kidney, Monkey kidney, Chick embryo, Chicken egg, Duck egg.
Calf (bovine) serum.
Betapropiolactone.
Foetal bovine serum.
Formaldehyde.
Formalin.
Gelatin.
Glycerol.
Human diploid cells (originating from human

aborted foetal tissue)
Hydrolyzed gelatin.
Monosodium glutamate.(MSG)
Neomycin.
Neomycin sulphate.
Phenol red indicator.
Phenoxyethanol.(antifreeze)
Potassium diphosphate
Potassium monophosphate.
Polymyxin B.
Polysorbate 20.
Polysorbate 80.
Porcine(pig)pancreatic hydrolysate of casein.
Residual MRC5proteins.
Sorbitol.
Sucrose.(sugar)
Thimerosal(49.6% mercury)
Tri(n)butylphosphate.
VERO cells, a continuous line of monkey kidney cells, washed sheep red blood cells.(10)

A famous American civil war general once said, **"Don't believe anything you hear & believe only half of what you see"**, in this case it sounds like good advice. P.S.Antibiotics are prone to destroying the good bacteria in our stomach, so if an antibiotic is required, Manuka honey (see article) or a natural herbal or fruit based one is the answer.

CHAPTER 11

VITAMINS & DISEASE

Make sure you are sitting down before you read this.

If you are of a sensitive or trusting nature, especially with regard to your Doctor or Oncologist the following paragraphs may be particularly distressing to read & I apologise if this is the case, But,. Nevertheless it needs to be said, however painful it may be, because it is the truth & you will not hear it from your Medical Practitioner, at least not voluntarily.

One of the commonest diseases associated with Diet,(although not always) & invariably Vitamin deficiency leading to Immune Deficiency (apart from stress) is **Cancer.** Wether you believe it to be Hereditary or otherwise is Immaterial.

It is one of the most feared & yet relatively one of the easiest of the major diseases to prevent & indeed cure, although you would never think this if the movie scripts & newspaper headlines are anything to go by ,The tear jerking sad films, like **Ali McGraw/Ryan Oneils"Love story"(1970) Danielle Steeles "Fine things"(1990) "No higher love"(1999) "Two against time"(2002)** to mention just a few of the multitudes of similar movies & soap operas with a terminal disease theme, usually Cancer, The Star almost always dies because this reflects the thinking of the general public,& judging by the Cancer Mortality rate I am not surprised, it would be unthinkable to have it any other way Could you imagine the Star being cured after all the build up, & the Doctors deadly diagnosis ?(& even more deadly treatment) When someone is diagnosed with cancer they are usually in shock when told & the natural reaction is to ask the Doctor "What do I do now"? the doctor of course recommends a course of Chemotherapy & /or Radiation therapy & /or surgery if necessary, its taken for granted that these are the only treatments available because no other treatments are ever mentioned, there is such a thing as "Non Destructive Chemotherapy" but this is not what is offered in the vast majority of cases because this is the type of Chemotherapy offered in Metabolic therapy clinics & is not the huge profit generating hard drugs normally used by most Oncologists, the public & most Cancer patients know only too well what to expect when they go for treatment, many friends & possibly relatives have trod the same road & many have never come back, it is this dismal failure rate in standard Cancer treatment that generates fear & the feeling that Cancer is a death sentence **when in fact it is not**, I know that sounds like heresy, but before you pass judgment on this statement take some time & approach it with a clear head & investigate the virtues of other more Natural treatments, Because in order to effect a cure for any disease, not just Cancer, you need a therapy that works in Harmony with the Immune system, **NOT AGAINST IT,** as Chemotherapy does,(Many Specialists say this, not just me) The Immune system is the bodies first line of defence against **all** disease & its integrity must be maintained at all costs, Its integrity & strength is maintained by Vitamins & minerals & numerous other nutrients, vitamins are used to fight & destroy diseases because they contain Enzymes & numerous other Antioxidants, Vitamin B17 is a vitamin not very widely known outside of Metabolic therapy circles, it has the ability to target & destroy rogue cells, This is why Metabolic Therapy in particular is such a versatile treatment for Cancer because it works **WITH** the bodies systems & complements the Immune system in particular & revitalizes the cells also, This is Natural healing as God intended & like all his other creations **IT WORKS,** (Contrary to what the so called "Specialists" will tell you)Why would it not work ? God himself designed it for this purpose,. Do you think the Specialists know better than God?

Laetrile is the chief anti tumour agent in B17 It is composed of 2 glucose molecules & 1 Benzaldehyde molecule with a Cyanide radical which is only formed in the presence of Betaglucosidase.

Betaglucosidase is an enzyme that only Cancer

cells have & this is the catalyst that activates the Hydrogen Cyanide molecule in Laetrile &together with the Benzaldehyde molecule initiates the destruction of the Cancer cell. The 2 glucose molecules are activated by Rhodanese & they proceed to nourish the healthy cells. Rhodanese is found in all healthy non cancerous cells.

The Hydrogen Cyanide molecule is not "Free floating", indeed it cannot neither exist or function without Betaglucosidase, if Rhodanese comes into contact with the Hydrogen Cyanide molecule it converts it into "**Thiocyanate**" thus rendering it harmless. **Bromelaine** (an enzyme found in raw Pineapples) also targets cancer cells & breaks down the protective shell cancer cells have, this leaves them vulnerable for Laetrile to do its thing, they work in partnership & complement each other, Is this not the Creator's handiwork ? & the best thing about this treatment is that when you are on it you feel like a million dollars because your body is being rejuvenated as well as being healed, have you ever known or seen Cancer patients in a Hospice or Hospital treatment centre looking or feeling like this? I think not, A word of warning may be appropriate here, If you decide to try Metabolic therapy as an alternative to conventional treatments do not expect your Doctor or Oncologist to be happy or complement your decision, very often their reaction can be quite hostile, you have bruised their ego & their pride.

As of August 2000 the United States food & drug administration (**FDA**) outlawed the sale or importation of vitaminB17,The growing or propagation of the Bitter Almond tree was also banned in 1995 (a very rich source of B17) also the **EU** in Brussels passed legislation(in 2007) to put all vitamins in the category of drugs & also restrict the dosage you can buy thus ensuring that B17 in tablet or capsule form will only be available by proscription & then only in small dosages,(rendering it useless for therapeutic purposes) all vitamins will also be under the control of the Pharmaceutical giants, Do you smell a rat here, you should, it's the Medical & Pharmaceutical industry restricting your choices of treatment & trying to make sure B17 Metabolic therapy is not one of the options, An example. of how desperate the Medical & Pharmaceutical profession is to maintain its hold on the cancer treatment market is an article in the **Daily Mail** (14/07/06) The story is about a 16 year old boy in the U.S.A. Abraham Cherrix (Virginia).who, after having horrendous side effects from Chemo treatment for Hodgkins disease, resolved never to have Chemo again, the boys parents got him onto a herbal based metabolic treatment, & were threatened with a charge of "medical neglect"& the Medical & Social services departments applied to get custody of the boy & **force** him to have another round of Chemo therapy, the boy said "I think it (chemotherapy) will kill me a second time"(on 21/07/06 the high court judge ruled in favour of the Medical & Social services to enforce chemotherapy treatment against the will of the boy & his parents) p.s. the boy was being treated with alternative treatments at a clinic in Mexico.

The "Oasis of Hope" Hospital in Tijuana, Mexico, founded by Dr. Ernesto Contreras has treated more than 100,000 Cancer patients, most of them very successfully with B17 Metabolic Therapy for the last 37 years, his Son Dr. Francisco Contreras is now the Director./Chief Surgeon.

Did you know that in the very liberal United Kingdom if your children are 16 years old or under & have been diagnosed with Cancer they can be forcibly taken from you & forcibly medicated with Chemotherapeutic drugs, & if you refuse to comply you can be imprisoned?...Believe it, it has already happened, & will continue as the Medical & Pharmaceutical professions become more desperate & more greedy & of course more unscrupulous. Cancer is not just a disease its an industry, It is a fact that there are more people employed in the Cancer industry than those who actually have Cancer.

Why would you want to even consider highly toxic drugs that not only destroy vital organs as well as your Immune system but make you constantly sick & feeling like you would rather be dead than endure any more, also the fact **(& it is a fact ,not a theory)** that most, if indeed not all of these Chemotherapeutic drugs **don't** work for your benefit in the long run, if they did the research labs. would not be constantly looking for new cures, you have heard the old adage "If it works don't fix it". The Cancer Research organizations are desperate to show they are actually achieving something in order to justify the huge donations & Government funding they get & the last thing they want is someone telling desperate people that they can be cured naturally & without nasty side effects, this is why you very rarely hear about natural treatments, can you imagine the nose dive the Chemo Drug market would take if Metabolic therapy was widely known & caught on, the vast majority of Cancer patients die from complications, usually repeated chest, or respiratory tract infections resulting from the immune system being destroyed, also other side effects of the Chemo drugs including organ failure & ultimately Heart failure rather than the Cancer itself, Not to mention the Psychological devastation of having your hair fall out in some cases, This does not help your self esteem, Drugs that make you feel & look sick cannot be doing you much good even though the doctors will tell you to stick with it (& they will tell you this with a straight face)

But this is not the worst indignity, Quite a few women (even some in their early 20,s) have had perfectly healthy breasts removed (total mastectomy) on the advice of their Oncologist as a precaution if there has been an incidence of breast Cancer in their family, very recently three women, who although they did not have Cancer consented to have their perfectly healthy breasts removed & also had Hysterectomies as a preventative measure because other members of their family & relatives had died of Cancer, the Oncologists said they had a defective gene & had an 80% chance of contracting Cancer,(10) Cancer cells are opportunistic, they are like Vagrants, they settle where the conditions are favourable & then begin to multiply, if the conditions are not favourable they cannot live or multiply, the answer is not to cut out organs but rather to make it impossible for these rogue cells to live & breed by boosting the Immune system with specific Immune boosting foods.

This form of totally unnecessary (as opposed to necessary) Surgery is legalized butchery to say the least, but alas, like many other questionable Medical procedures it is legal.& the patients agree to it, Such is the persuasive power of these Medical Gurus & the fear generated in their trusting patients, It is truly amazing how well the Medical

& Pharmaceutical industry have succeeded in eliminating all traces of Natural therapies that are of any major threat to them, they have managed (mostly by manipulation or bribes) to keep these Therapies out of the Media spotlight & distract the public attention by Hyping up the latest Drug breakthrough, they have been doing this for close on 70 years now, they are masters in the art of Deception & money is no object in maintaining their deceit.(remember the quotation by George Orwell at the beginning of this book).October 2007 is Breast Cancer awareness month, "Think pink"is the slogan you will hear to boost breast cancer awareness & promote the numerous cancer societies. It is very interesting that Vitamin D either in tablet or sunlight form can prevent up to 77% of all cancers including the common breast & colon cancers but yet the Cancer societies & Institutes will not promote this amazing cure, did you ever wonder why?

The answer is simple, Detection makes money, Prevention loses it! This is why millions of dollars/pounds is invested in Scanners & other expensive detection machines & so little is invested in Prevention, in the context of the very cosy relationship between the Cancer societies & the Pharmaceutical conglomerates Prevention is definitely not better than cure (or more accurately "Treatment") it is by no means as lucrative, the drug manufacturers depend on people getting cancer to make their obscenely vast profits, preventitative measures would vastly reduce those profits, this is why the Cancer industry is the biggest money spinner of all time, Did you know that an estimated 600,000 cases of Breast & Colorectal cancer could be saved by a daily intake of vitamin D3,the cancer societies & leading oncologists know all this but they will not tell their patients because they know their career is at stake if they do, such is the deceit which has caused the demise of even the rich & famous, many of which were & still are allowed to die on the alter of expediency to protect the sacred cows of the medical & pharmaceutical drug pushers…**Money & Power!**

.Look at it another way, If you are a Christian & your body is the Temple of the Holy Ghost why would you allow it to be desecrated or mutilated & eventually killed off (if you have enough Chemo or Radiation sessions) when you could treat the disease naturally as God intended (.Or if you eat right you will not get the disease in the first place, even if your whole family has had it). Needless to say Natural therapies are discouraged & frowned upon by the orthodox medical Establishment, not because they do not work but because they are a threat to their lucrative incomes, not to mention their ego's.

If you have, or had been diagnosed with cancer, when did your Doctor, or Oncologist ever ask you what your primary diet preferences were? eg.- what foods or meats you ate & how often & how much in an effort to ascertain what caused your Cancer? they will rarely ask you these questions because they are totally drug orientated & most have a very limited knowledge of nutrition & its virtues (or the consequences of poor nutrition), Poor nutrition is not confined to those on low incomes or Senior Citizens you can be filthy rich & still live on poorly nutritious junk food, **The American Cancer Society** in a statement in 1994 called "Cancer facts and figures" said,--**"More than $104 billion is spent on cancer ,including** treatment, lost productivity & mortality costs.(the cost of dying) One third of the annual 500,000 deaths from cancer, including Breast, Colon, & Prostate cancers, may be attributed to "UNDESIRABLE DIETARY PRACTICES",(SO WHY DONT THEY ASK YOU WHAT YOUR DIETARY PRACTICES ARE?)Is that too much to ask? It is if you know little or nothing about Nutrition. or the effects of poor nutrition.

It is interesting to note that a questionnaire given to 118 cancer Doctors at the **McGill** University Cancer centre in Montreal Canada revealed that 79 Doctors responded, of which 64 said they would not consent to be part of any trial involving Cisplatin (one of the commonest drugs of 6 being trialled) 58 of the 64 said they would not consent to any of the 6 trials due to the **"Ineffectiveness of Chemotherapy & its unacceptably high degree of Toxicity"** Can you beat that for hypocrisy? These people are asking you to trust their judgment & accept chemotherapeutic drugs they would not touch with a bargepole, if they were in your position.

Chemo drugs can only be given for short periods because this sustained assault on the body can only be tolerated by the organs for so long, then they pack up, Do you actually believe your Doctor when he tells you this is a beneficial treatment?(**73%of Doctors polled in the U.S.A.don't think so**), A study of chemo drugs by a team of scientists at the University of Rochester[U.S.A 30/11/06.] led by DR.Joerg Dietrich, found that some of the principal drugs used in chemotherapy may damage healthy brain cells more than the cancer cells they are meant to target, the drugs used to treat Breast & Lung cancer as well as Leukaemia kill some types of brain cells as well as hampering others from dividing, some cancer patients treated with Chemotherapy have shown a marked reduction in Cognitive abilities, The research, published in the" Journal of Biology "charts the effects of chemo drugs **CISPLATIN,** which is used to treat Breast, Lung, & Colon cancer,..**CARMUSTINE,** used for Brain tumours & Hodgkin's disease, & **CYTARABINE,** used to treat Leukaemia,. **CISPLATIN is officially a Class 2 Carcinogen** (cancer causing agent) & all containers of this drug require a label indicating it is Poisonous &

Corrosive, Boy, does that ever take your breath away! It could, LITERALLY!

Some of the drugs that were used 40 years ago to treat Cancer were suspended by the government because too many patients were dying from the side effects.

,**A Z T**was one of these & it is still listed in the **British Pharmacopoeia & Mims (Pharmaceutical drug reference catalogues).**& still used as a treatment for **A.I.D.S.,** Dr.Mohammed Ali Al Bayati (PhD. D.A.B.T..D.A.B.V.T).Toxicologist & Pathologist, said many of the side effects of A.Z.T. actually mimic A.I.D.S.symptoms, Some of the side effects of A.Z.T.are eg.—

Severe bone marrow depression.

Reduction in white cell count.inc.**T** cells (Remember the **T** cells in chapter 9)

Very toxic to stem cells in bone marrow.

Widespread Systemic damage to Liver, Kidneys, Pancreas,& other organs.

This is just one of the treatments inflicted on unsuspecting A.I.D.S.patients. These drugs were reintroduced again in recent years to treat A.ID,s patients in Africa, needless to say they died like flies (& still do), in most cases it is not AIDs that is wrong with them but rather **Malnutrition, & Dysentery,** the commonest causes of death in Africa in all generations, Do you remember the massive AIDS publicity surrounding the Gays & Junkies of the 60s & 70s in the U.K. but only a small fraction of them had AIDs, it was **Malnutrition** compounded by booze & drugs & very little sleep because of their continuous parties that gave the appearance & symptoms of AIDs, even the blood samples were contaminated with drugs in many cases & as always it was misdiagnosed, they were given Chemotherapy which weakened their already weakened bodies even more & killed off their immune system (what was left of it) very few, if any, ever survived this onslaught of medical science.

,**PS** ...Please allow me to let you into a secret which even many Doctors don't know, **H.I.V.** is supposedly a virus **(Retrovirus)** which leads to, or causes **A.I.D.**s, The amazing thing is that no Culture or even a tangible, visible Virus has ever been isolated or proven to exist either in laboratories or elsewhere, Dr.Eleni Papadopulos Ph.D. Professor of Medical Physics (Perth) & many others have supported this view.

Dr.Mohammed Ali Al Bayati has also said, "Get all the facts, H.I.V. does not cause A.I.D.S."

You should also be aware how easy it is to be mistakenly diagnosed with H.I.V.

There are over 60 medical conditions, from which the blood tests can mistakenly indicate a so called H.I.V.infection, This conclusion is arrived at when a blood test indicates raised antibody activity (this only indicates that the immune system is fighting bugs, it could be any one of millions) neither these routine tests or specific H.I.V.tests indicate Viral activity, Even the Drug companies who manufacture the test kits admit this.

Some of the 60+conditions which have been misdiagnosed in the past (& the present) as being H.I.V. positive are...
FLU (Including the Flu jab)
TETANUS (Including the Tetanus jab)
MALARIA

HEPATITIS A & B (Including the Hepatitis jab)
HAEMOPHILIA
ORGAN TRANSPLANT
RENAL FAILURE
VIRAL INFECTIONS
ALCOHOL & DRUG USE
PREGNANCY

So called "H.I.V. POSITIVE" blood test readings carry little or no Diagnostic value & this is fast becoming known as the greatest medical fraud of the 20th.& 21st.century.

$20,000 or £10,000 has been offered to anyone who can prove the existence of the so called H.I.V.virus, No one has claimed this prize in the last 20 years, Obviously today's Doctors or Scientists either don't need this kind of money, or else the more logical conclusion is that they cannot substantiate their claims of the existence of an H.I.V. virus, Is this not a logical conclusion?

While on the subject of Vitamins & Disease you may be interested, or indeed even surprised to know some interesting things about **"Vitamin D"**,It is a scientific fact that the length of your ring finger can be a strong indicator of your chances of developing Heart disease by your mid 30s if you are a male, Your ring finger should be at least 2%longer than your index finger, during the critical development stage Genes that affect Testosterone production also determine the length of finger development, Hormone concentrations are dependant on certain Vitamin levels & a deficiency of Vitamin D can mean a reduction in Testosterone levels which in turn can potentially increase your chances of Heart problems by your mid 30,s.

But this does not mean you have to sit around & wait for a heart attack or heart disease, you can beat the system by adopting a healthy lifestyle & increasing your intake of vitamin "D" the most effective way is by getting more sun (Sunlight converts "Sterols" on your skin to vitamin D) or fruits or Veg. with a high vitamin D content.

Another dramatic discovery is that a very concentrated dosage of vitamin D, 4,000 IU (International Units) daily can demonstrate a significant improvement in patients with Parkinson's disease.

Also of major interest is another development in

the treatment of Cancer, recent tests showed that those women with the highest blood levels of vitamin D3 had the lowest risk of Breast Cancer & conversely those with the lowest blood levels of vitamin D had the highest risk of Breast Cancer.

Raising the levels of vitamin D in the blood from 26ng/ml. to 34ng/ml. was shown to reduce the rate of colorectal cancer by half & an increase in blood levels to 46ng/ml further reduced the risk factor by two thirds.

2,000 IU of Vit. D3 daily reduces Breast Cancer by 50%(Dept.of family & preventative medicine, University of California, San Diego)(12)

Do you remember the history of **SCURVY** the dreaded disease British sailors were prone to, according to naval records over **1,000,000** sailors died of scurvy between 1600 -1800, yet for hundreds of years the cure for this awful disease had already been part of the official record, Sir Richard Hawkins & other notable seamen discovered that eating Limes & Lemons & other Citrus fruits cured Scurvy very quickly, because this was essentially a "Vitamin C" deficiency but the Medical fraternity was not interested in hearing what Sir Richard had to say, not because they could not understand or see the relevance of all these facts but more than likely because they saw this fruit based cure as a threat to their credibility, especially as it was a non medical person who recognized this cure, in addition to this these medical gurus of the day stood to lose money, not to mention prestige if people rejected conventional medicines in favour of fruit based cures, These Doctors were held in very high esteem & when the Admiralty chiefs consulted with them about this alleged cure for Scurvy they acted on their advice because of their status as Doctors & done precisely nothing, It was the Pride of these Doctors that killed the millions of Scurvy victims, not just the scurvy itself, needless to say it is still pride that kills the millions of disease victims around the world, & especially in the so called "Western Civilized Society" where it is sometimes harder to stay alive and well than it would be in the middle of the Amazon jungle.

By the time of the Napoleonic wars more British soldiers were dying from Ascorbic acid (VIT. C) deficiency(scurvy) than were being killed in combat, all this because the Medical establishment did not wish to recognize any cure which did not involve drugs, it took 450 years & millions of deaths before the vitamin C treatment became official naval policy.

B17metabolic therapy has been known widely in medical & scientific circles for more than 70 years, but very little if anything is ever heard about it, indeed most people, including Health food shops don't even know what B17is,why is this? Why has this therapy which has cured many thousands of lives never been publicised or offered as an alternative treatment? the answer is simple, Metabolic therapy is a Natural Fruit based treatment & because it occurs in nature it cannot be patented, so, **no patent, no profit**, also because the root cause of the disease is cured there is no need for repeat proscriptions, This would not be good news for the drug companies, whose aim is to alleviate the symptoms of diseases not cure them, also the fact that many top medical Consultants are on the board of directors of some of the biggest drug companies & Chemo manufacturers, Metabolic therapy would not be on their list of priorities.

Now you know that it is in your best interests to get healthy & stay healthy, so if you are diagnosed as having cancer & your consultant recommends chemo, ask him if he would take it if he had cancer, his answer might surprise you, (if he is honest that is),Its an interesting fact that if you elected to accept no treatment at all & continue living as normal you would live 4 times longer than you would if you accepted conventional treatments,- eg,- chemo or radiation therapy. (This is fact & attested to by the worlds leading Oncologists)But will our medical wizards accept Gods remedies & admit that he knows best? Not while there is a huge financial incentive for them to think otherwise, the relevance of Gods laws for the Christian & non Christian alike is even more applicable now than ever before, the Devil conceals or distorts the truth of Gods word, this is why we need to be informed so we will not be hoodwinked & believe the big lie, "Hath God said"? yes God has said, the trouble Is when it comes to health & obedience issues many of Gods Ministers are not saying, either because they are as guilty as their flock or because they do not wish to cause offence, knowing as they obviously do that most of their congregations are guilty of breaking Gods laws mainly through ignorance rather than just plain disobedience.

The Metabolic Therapy mentioned in this chapter & others is still administered & studied at the world famous "Oasis of Hope" Hospital in Tijuana, Mexico, also Metabolic therapy courses & day treatment centres are available as well as long stay facilities, Individual Metabolic therapy components can also be bought there, contact them on the internet www.oasisofhope.com. Also in the U.K."Credence Publications" can advise & sell Metabolic Therapy components.—(Tabs. Capsules, B17injections, Apricot seeds, related books etc.--) also a list of Doctors willing to give Metabolic Therapy treatment privately on an outpatient basis both in Ireland (North & South) & the U.K contact www.credencepublications.co (Philip Day)

CHAPTER 12

GLUTTONY, THE COMMONEST SIN

It is probably one of the commonest, if indeed not the commonest sin in Christendom primarily I believe because Christians do not see it as a sin indeed most indulge in it without even thinking about it, its almost second nature.

Solomon knew the down side of it when he said, "Put a knife to thy throat if thou be a man given to appetite"(Proverbs 23-2) When we see an alcoholic or drunkard in the street we almost look down on them like a lower form of life, or like the Levite, pass by on the other side, but in actual fact Alcoholism is really no worse than Gluttony in some respects both are equally as bad, while the Alcoholic may inevitably drink himself to death, the Glutton invariably eats him, or herself to death, they dig their grave with their fork.

I know very well it is not the done thing to speak

on the subject of diet, People are very sensitive about these subjects, they do not like to be told what is right to eat & what is not, so they remain in ignorance (in many cases wilfully) and pain, nevertheless this does not absolve the Christian from studying the scriptures for themselves, Paul the apostle instructed Timothy (2nd Timothy 2:15) "Study to show thyself approved unto God". You have an obligation to God and also to yourself to "Prove all things" (1st Thess 5:21). Many Christians **"Live to eat"** not eat to live, this is not just overeating or the occasional overindulgence, this is **"Gluttony"**,

GLUTTONY IS NOT ONLY A SIN, IT IS A DESECRATION OF THE TEMPLE OF GOD! "Know ye not that ye are not your own for ye are bought with a price, therefore glorify God in your body,& in your spirit which are Gods" (1 st. Corinthians 6..19-20) Our bodies are the temple of God but if the temple of old was maintained like we maintain our bodies the maintenance men would have been stoned, poor maintenance of our bodies is like the m.o.t. on a car, an inspector would never pass it, neither does

God pass it when Gluttons constantly over indulge & put their bodies systems in turmoil this is why they are constantly sick & plagued with physical problems,

Obesity is a symptom of Gluttony (& usually inactivity) & can be the root cause of numerous problems not the least being **Heart problems, Coronary Artery Disease, High blood pressure, Circulatory problems, Renal problems, Osteoarthritis, Gout, Gallbladder disease, Diabetes,** to name but a few, (80% with type 2 diabetes are Obese) There is also an increased risk of **Breast, Endometrial, or Colon Cancer, as well as lower back pain.**

One of the less known factors which contribute to Obesity is SLEEP or more precisely the lack of it, there is a Hormone called **"LEPTIN"** & this can become dysfunctional if you do not get the proper amount of sleep, when this happens it sends messages to the brain, which in turn affects the burn rate of your fat reserves.

LEPTIN also plays a significant or even primary role in **Heart disease,. Osteoporosis,. Autoimmune disease,.Reproductive diseases,**

& even the rate of Ageing.(13)

One of the things I have noticed is that Obese people are **not** prone to doing nothing about their problem , indeed many are very positive about it & do appear to be keen to do something, anything, EXCEPT EAT LESS....Many have surgery to get their Stomach stapled, or others have a Gastric Band fitted to restrict their intake of solids, pureed food is all they can take, but many cannot stick the course & quit because of a restricted diet & sickness, while others have surgery to have mounds of excess flab cut away or others have surgery to have internal fat suctioned away (Liposuction),Why do they put themselves through this purgatory when all they have to do is adopt a proper dietary regime (see ch.22) & eat sensibly,& adapt their food consumption level to suit their needs, & get the job done, they don't have to starve, just eat less,& eat the right kind of foods & eventually they will get there, their stomach will shrink as they eat less & they will get used to small meals, **ALSO ,DO NOT FORGET TO EXERCISE** not just a walk in the park but a proper Gym based all round Planned routine, This may sound like a bad word but it is ESSENTIAL, the two go hand in hand.

What a poor state of affairs this is,because not only can Gods people not control their fork,they indulge in the worst kind of food,e.g. pastries ,ice cream, sugary drinks, fizzy drinks, (most of which contain a high level of Aspartame) greasy foods, saturated fats,eg.—fat coated foods designed for oven cooking,fatty meat (instead of lean meat) Many people have told me,its in their genes or they just cannot reduce because their body assimilates fat too easily, or they put it on too easily, HOGWASH, Apart from steroids which some people may have trouble with,these are not valid excuses for being obese,Did you ever see an obese or over weight prisoner of war? certainly not, because its not only what you eat that counts but how much, gluttons eat like they do because their love of food comes before their general health, or love of God, they are not committed to doing Gods will when they unashamedly flout Gods laws that were given specifically to keep them healthy to serve him, Philippians 3 -19 says **"Their god is their belly"**Solomon also classed gluttons alongside drunkards "The drunkard & the glutton shall come to poverty"(Proverbs 23-21) ,no matter what the "Big is beautiful" brigade says "Big" is unhealthy & they know it, tried all the slimming diets & nothing works? Try Gods diet, it works, if you work it, an old quotation I learned many years ago in the sales business, "Its easy if you work it hard, but hard if you try to work it easy" applies to the food laws, knowing what to eat, how much to eat & when to eat it, is the key to success.

I & many nutritionists have long since proved that little & often is the key to excellent health, this would normally be 5-6 small meals per day (& I do mean small) this allows the bodies digestive system to assimilate& digest food without putting undue stress on it, it also helps to control the stomachs gastric juices because the less the stomach has to handle the less Hydrochloric acid is required to break down the food mass ,over production of gastric juices causes indigestion, heartburn ,& stomach ulcers,& what of the famous old "Ulster fry"? forget it,the old adage, "A good breakfast sets you up for the day" is bunkum, it was probably a glutton who said that, breakfast should be light, because your body is still in the elimination cycle & not set up for a lot of work at this time of the day, Tea or fruit juice should not be taken with any meal unless absolutely necessary& then only small sips, any fluid taken with a meal dilutes the stomachs gastric juices & makes the digestion process longer, & the stomachs work harder, no wonder you have "Indigestion" if you must take a drink be it Tea, Juice, or whatever allow ½ hour at least for your meal to digest, then drink.

The body operates on 3 main cycles over 24 hours eg…

Noon till 8 pm is the appropriation cycle when your body is most receptive for its fuel intake, it is important to eat only when your body is hungry… Not You!

8 pm until 4 am is the Assimilation cycle, This occurs mostly at night & ideally must run on time, this is the period when all the food you have eaten during the day is sifted & broken down into its molecular substances & all the proteins,, minerals &,vitamins are extracted from it & transported via the 10,000 miles of arteries & blood vessels the body is supplied with,**Night time** (usually from 8pm on) is not a good time to eat because the body is resting & this is the ideal time for the digestive system to get cranked up & do its thing with the minimum of disruption, the system works best when we are at rest & if you leave 3 hours between your last meal & when you go to bed by the time you lay your head on the pillow your supper will be well on its way through the digestive system & the nutrients extracted from it, then it (provided its not nutrient deficient junk food) will be in the process of being extracted & distributed throughout the body, replenishing damaged cells & allowing the blood & lymphatic systems to pick up the waste & take it to the garbage collection points in preparation for elimination the following morning, if however you decide to wolf down a pizza or something similar just prior to going to bed, your body ,being in a horizontal position & gravity working against your stomach will make you feel like you have eaten a horse & the Hydrochloric acid reflux in your stomach will demand a bucket of antacids to cool down ,but as always the systems operate best when they are not over loaded & there are plenty of nutrients to keep it ticking over like a Swiss watch.

4am till 12 Noon is the Elimination cycle when the body's waste is ready to be discharged, all the food debris & other junk that cannot be absorbed or utilised is assembled for collection & disposal via the numerous outlets, the body has very efficient methods of disposing of its waste as well as metabolic toxins, Toxins are shunted out via the lymphatic system through the Underarm glands The glands on the back of the knees, glands behind the Ears , Groin ,Nose, Mouth , & the Skin , If you clog up the pores with deodorants this also prevents the elimination of toxins from some lymphatic outlets & can cause a build up of toxins in that area,many of these deodorants have toxic metals in their ingredients & a good wash is just as good,(14) If you had a Pristine expensive car you would not put cheap oil in the engine ,because it is finely engineered & tuned it requires the best oil available ,cheap oil will eventually degenerate into a gooey sludge & gum up the engine your body is worth a lot more than an expensive car & is far more intricate & technologically advanced than any machine & it requires superior nutrients to keep it in pristine condition, cheap fast foods & devitalized cereals & supermarket specials are a sure remedy for disaster.

Many Christians are the authors of their own destruction because they fail to observe the fact that they are wilfully sinning on a daily basis through their eating habits, although to be fair it is also true to say that many are not aware of this because of ignorance through lack of instruction & to those in this latter category you can now say you have been instructed & as of now you are without excuse.

CHAPTER 13

THE UNCLEAN MEATS

Untold agony & disease results from the consumption of unclean meats there are numerous animals classed as unclean by god ,but by far the most infamous as well as the most toxic animal is the **SWINE**,more commonly known as the

PIG, or HOG, the pig is a scavenger,& as such it feeds on virtually all manner of dead or dying flesh even the bodies of other pigs, not to mention the putrid sores & cancerous tissue of other dead animals which die on the same farm,apart from rotting vegetables & other swill, Why is the pig so potently poisonous? Primarily because of its digestive system which is relatively primitive & very simple, the pigs digestive system is so plain & straightforward that whatever it eats is through its stomach & intestines & absorbed into its tissues in just 4 hours, there is virtually no filtering of toxins or separation of toxic substances so that whatever the animal was eating prior to being slaughtered is already in its cells & is passed on to the customer in the Pork, Ham, Bacon,ect.

This is in contrast to cows, they have 3 stomachs & the food is filtered & detoxified through these stomachs, also it is not a scavenger or meat eater.

London's eminent scientist, Sir James Paget said of the pig, "Fancy the body of a single individual supporting more separately existing creatures than the whole population of the world". Seem impossible? Dr. Maurice c.Hall,chief of the division of Zoology of the U.S. public Health service commented "It appears to be a legitimate demand that when a man exchanges dollars for Pork, he should not do it on the basis that he may be purchasing his death warrant", this was his comment on the pig.

And what of the subtle killer **TRICHINOSIS,** found in other animals but the most willing host & by far the most infested with this disease is the good old Pig again, This disease originates with the Trichina worm ,just one of about 18 or19 different worms found in the flesh of pigs ,but none as deadly as the Trichina, so minute & transparent are these worms they are almost undetectable, but their effect on the body is not so undetectable, because you can feel its presence in the multitude of ailments attributable to it, the biggest problem is linking these ailments to the worm ,Physicians have confused trichnosis with at least 50 other ailments ranging from Typhoid fever to alcoholism ,this extremely toxic worm is so hard to detect & so good at staying alive even when tested under extreme heat, that it's the ultimate survivor, and killer, in autopsies the trichnea worm is never looked for so it is never found unless by accident, but for those coroners who are observant enough to inspect the bodies more thoroughly it can be more revealing, a Dr. Manley, an expert on animal diseases made the statement that autopsies showed that 1 in every 3 people are infected with Trichinosis, I don't need to tell you what this means, do I? It is interesting to note that the Hebrew name for "Abominable" is **PIGGUL**, this is where the name PIG comes from.

The Prophet Isaiah prophesied the words of God & said **"I have spread out my hands all the day unto a rebellious people…A people that provoketh me to anger continually to my face…..Which eat Swines flesh & broth of abominable things, Behold it is written before me, I will not keep silence but will recompense, even recompense into their bosom."(Isaiah 65-2)** This is a prophecy concerning ancient Israel's rebellious ways but I feel it is equally applicable to us in this generation, God was incensed because of Israel's defiant attitude to his laws, the attitude of many Christians today is equally defiant &

it is obvious they are paying the price for it in Disease.

When the Prophet said **"I will recompense into their bosom"**, I thought to myself, How common is **Bowel cancer, Colon cancer, Intestinal cancer, Cervical cancer, Endometrial (womb) cancer, Pancreatic cancer,** These are principal Cancers in the Abdominal area & are among the most common in Men & Women & would appear to be most commonly associated with **DIET,** Does all this say something to you, if you are thinking logically, it should, this is the price you could be paying if you deviate from Gods Law & do your own thing, Disease is no respecter of persons & makes no distinction between Believers or Unbelievers, Examine your diet, because contrary to what the so called experts may tell you, This is where it all begins, it all comes back to the Universal law of Cause & Effect **"For every effect there is a cause"** every disease has its origin in the food we eat or the fluid we drink, or the environment we inhabit or work in, The pig was created to be a scavenger, as was the Vulture ,& numerous other creatures both small &

large, scavengers were designed to clean up dead carcasses & other putrefying dead matter in order to reduce widespread infection & disease, they were designed to serve humanity in this capacity, they were NEVER meant to be eaten by Humans.

CHAPTER 14

SOME OBJECTIONS

There are those who would argue that God has done away with the food laws & we are no longer bound by them, Let me ask a question, did the New Testament saints keep the food laws? Did the early church keep them? We are in the new Dispensation the same as the early church, so if they believed & taught it then we are duty bound to do so also,...sadly many have departed from the faith once delivered to the saints & they quote Paul the Apostle to support their departure, (1 Timothy Ch. 4-v3)"Forbidding to marry & commanding to abstain from meats which God hath created to be received with thanksgiving of them which believe & know the truth", The Greek rendering of this is **"Which God hath created for reception"**, God did not create EVERYTHING for reception, otherwise everything would be quite edible, including, Cockroaches, Rats, Snakes, Spiders, indeed just about every creepy crawly, including Dogs & Cats (That's strange, why don't we see Dog meat or Cat meat in the butchers ,or Tarantula legs) Verse 4 states "For every creature of God is good & nothing to be refused if it be received with thanksgiving", Does this mean any thing & every thing whether it be the nastiest creepy crawlies or the filthiest hog is good to eat, does it mean God has transformed previously unclean creatures into clean ones & made them o.k. to eat? I think not! This is a question of Interpretation of the term "Creature of God"(v.4) The verse does not say "Every creature that God created", it says "Every creature of God", there is a big difference, the Bible does not contradict itself, Every creature of God means Every creature that God has deemed suitable for human consumption, creatures that will not be a threat to our health, Why would God deem certain creatures Unclean in the Old

Testament & then change his mind & permit their consumption in the New Testament,? are these animals any different now, than they were then? Of course they are not, the key to the interpretation of this verse is," Every creature of God is good", but not every creature that God created, because this would include the unclean creatures as well as the clean ones.

CHAPTER 15

THE EATING OF BLOOD

It is only natural that you should be shocked by this statement, I know what you are thinking, "Eat blood, sounds horrible, who would do such a thing, apart from an animal that is" well the fact is unless you are a strict vegetarian, you do, assuming that is, you eat red meat which almost everyone does, you don't need to be a genius to know that red meat is red because of the blood in it ,& whether you cook it, grill it, fry it, or stew it, it is still full of blood, the blood may be thickened or coagulated because of the cooking process but its still there, blood also putrefies more rapidly than muscle or fat or flesh, so you are still eating blood, wether its in a hamburger or worse still the dreaded black pudding or black sausage which is made mostly of blood (usually pigs blood, the worst of the worst)The bible tells us that the life is in the blood "For the life of the flesh is in the blood" (liviticus 17 -11), & also that it was Gods command to abstain from eating it (Leviticus 17 -10), "And whatsoever man there be of the house of Israel or of the strangers that sojourn among you that eateath any manner of blood, I will even set my face against that soul that eateth blood & will cut him off from among his people" This command was not only confined to the Israelites in their time, but was meant to be a guide for all generations in all times, the new testament also teaches the abstinence of blood consumption (Acts 15 – 29)" **That ye abstain from meats offered to idols & FROM BLOOD& from things strangled"**(ps-This does not refer to blood transfusions but rather meats of various kinds, I don't think medical science was that far advanced in Pauls day so he could not have known about this procedure) Not only is the life in the blood ,toxins are also present,-e.g.,-...growth hormones, vaccines, parasites & numerous other diseases carried via the blood.

It was very popular years ago for body builders to eat a lot of meat, usually as rare as possible, in the belief that it provided extra strength & muscle building qualities, this belief came about because carnivores in the wild especially Lions & Tigers were observed to gain a lot of muscle & strength from eating raw meat (from their prey) & the theory was if humans ate the same type of diet they would also make big muscular gains ,there is only one problem, Lions & Tigers & most other carnivores have specific enzymes which we do not have, these are designed to absorb & filter the various vitamins & minerals from raw meat& utilize them in their bodies also their digestive system is simpler & more adapted to the digestion of meat, their gastric juices are 20 times more powerful than ours so that meat can be broken down & absorbed into the system more easily, & quickly. Because meat putrefies so quickly the digestive system in carnivores is designed to process the meat quickly & eliminate it via the waste system before the putrefying process begins, this is achieved by a relatively short intestinal system the total length being only 3 times the length of the animal (convoluted & compressed into the abdominal cavity), as opposed to a much longer length in humans, humans are not carnivores & were not designed to eat meat, at least not raw meat anyway, meat has to be cooked or grilled & this destroys much of the nutritional value, also unlike the carnivores meat, supermarket meat is not guaranteed to be toxin free, Lions & Tigers usually only eat meat that they have just killed & it is generally healthy otherwise it could not give the big cats a run for their money also they have not been polluted with vaccines or other numerous injected hormones, it is also interesting to note that they generally only eat live animals, animals that they have killed themselves they rarely eat dead animals that have been lying for a while unless they are desperate, they also seem to know if an animal has died from disease or just old age, it seems when it comes to food, most animals are a lot wiser than we are. If meat is desired at least it should be drained of its blood, this is relatively simple, e.g. soak the meat in boiling water for ½ hour ,drain off the blood & salt it thoroughly for another ½ hour then drain & wash off the salt,(the salt draws out the remaining blood) ,at least now it is more or less fit to eat,.(or at least , fitter than it was before) The bible does not condemn the eating of meat ,provided it is clean (in the biblical sense that is) and its blood content is flushed out, although it is fair to say that not all meat is contaminated ,but there is always a risk involved, a risk that need not be taken, if the simple guidelines are followed, as stated above. It is interesting to note that scientists from the Medical Research Council in 2005 led by Professor Sheila Bingham (Cambridge) found a specific Cancer risk link with red meat which they classed as **Beef--Lamb--Pork--Veal**, they studied the diets of 500,000 men & women across Europe, they found that those who ate more than **51/2oz.(156 gr.)** of red meat per day were a third more likely to get Bowel Cancer,51/2 oz.would be the equivalent of,--A burger & 2 sausages, or--2 Lamb chops, or—3Cumberland sausages,-or-1 Pork loin steak-or-1Veal escalope,-or-1 rasher of Bacon& 2 pork sausages,-or-1 Lamb kebab,& the risk goes up even more when you eat 7 oz. or more of red meat per day, Is this not a good enough case for bloodless meat, Or indeed any meat, whether bloodless or not, once it is grilled or fried there is not a lot of nutrients left in it anyway.

CHAPTER 16

THE EATING OF FAT.

I was more than surprised when I learned how common the eating of fat really was, I found it hard to believe that anyone could actually like fat, & I don't mean the invisible fat that is present in most supermarket products like cereals, crisps, oven chips etc. I mean visible fat found on steaks, bacon, ribs, chicken etc. how can civilized people actually like that stuff? Worse still, how can they eat it? I can understand wild animals eating fat to boost their fat reserves for their winter insulation or hibernation, but humans? God warned the Israelites about the eating of fat because he knew how lethal it was, Leviticus ch.3-17 "It shall be a perpetual statute for your generations throughout all your dwellings, that you eat neither Fat nor Blood"

How much plainer can you get than that!! You don't need me to tell you that Coronary Artery disease is very prevalent, this comes about when fatty deposits clog the arteries & restrict the blood flow, or worse still,. block the blood flow altogether causing a heart attack, if this is the case no amount of C.P.R.,or defibrillation will restart your heart again, its stopped for good.

There are 3 main types of fat namely
POLYUNSATURATED FATS
SATURATED FATS
MONOUNSATURATED FATS

POLYUNSATURATED FATS
Found in **Oily fish Cooking oils e.g. Safflower oil, Grapeseed oil—Sunflower & corn oils— Low fat spreads** (not margarine, or butter)

These fats are by far the safest & are also necessary for healthy skin & the development of body cells, there are several types of polyunsaturates but the best types are those with a high concentration of **OMEGA 3,EFA,s** (Essential Fatty Acids) these are found in **Flax oil, Hemp oil, Pumpkin seeds, Walnuts & Oily fish.**

SATURATED FATS

Sources… Meats, Dairy products, Coconut oil & Hard cheeses.

Virtually all foods have some percentage of fat, some higher than others but not all fat is bad, of the three types mentioned above Saturated fats are by far the worst in terms of healthy eating ,Saturated fats are covered in Hydrogen atoms & tend to become deposited on the walls of arteries, this type of fat is solid, hard fat, & remains solid at room temperature & when it becomes lodged in arteries it hardens the arteries & they lose their elasticity, this leads to hardened arteries & through time they become blocked, if the victim survives the resultant heart attack (assuming his coronary arteries are affected) he will require a bypass operation or an artery graft (cutting out the blocked section & grafting on a new section,) An **Atherectomy** (shaving or lasering the artery walls to remove plaque) may also be an alternative, if the arteries in the head are affected a form of dementia, or a stroke could occur due to a reduction of oxygen to the brain.sometimes the Femoral arteries in the legs become so badly blocked that the blood supply is reduced to a trickle & gangrene can result, necessitating amputation of the limb, the same can happen to any limb.

High blood pressure & High Cholesterol are also side effects of a diet ,high in saturated fats, this can be the price you pay for dietary negligence & disobedience to the laws of God which are designed to keep you healthy…..P.S. the combination of Cholesterol &Saturated fat is known as Plaque.

MONOUNSATURATED FATS
Sources are. **Olive oil, Rapeseed oil, Hazelnuts, Almonds, Brazil nuts, Cashew nuts, Sesame seeds.** Extra Virgin Olive oil is the best oil for cooking, it also helps boost the immune system.

Mono fats are also believed to offer protection against Breast & Colon cancers.

POLYUNSATURATED & MONOUNSATURATED FATS are not

manufactured by the body but are essential for its health & maintenance, & are utilized by the body for Insulation (to help regulate temperature etc..--) They also act as Shock absorbers & Padding as well as bedding for the Internal Organs ect.—

As you see fat is essential for the health of the body, but only certain types are permitted to be eaten, Saturated fats are not.

CHAPTER 17

OUR FURRY FRIENDS
PETS & PET FOOD.

Just like their ancestors & present day cousins **Cats & Dogs are basically wild creatures**, Dogs may be more trainable & easier to domesticate than Cats but both are designed to live & thrive on **raw food** rather than cooked food, unlike most dogs, cats are hunters & in the wild do not cook their food, their teeth are like Tigers & all other carnivores, they are designed to rip & chew meat & crush bone, most cats & dogs do **not** thrive on commercial or cooked pet foods, (although they may seem to do)their systems are designed to assimilate & digest **RAW** food primarily meats, eg, **chicken, beef, liver, heart vegetables, grass** (for hairballs), commercial pet foods are not good nor designed for pets (contrary to what commercial manufacturers may say) ,Cats & dogs, contrary to popular opinion do not thrive on them for the simple reason, **cooked food is dead,** most of the nutrients & virtually all of the important enzymes present in raw meats is missing, killed by the cooking process, the amount of nutrients a healthy cat or dog needs to meet their daily requirements is not present in these pet foods, it is virtually impossible to manufacture any kind of pet food with all the basic nutritional ingredients in adequate amounts for the price you pay in super markets or pet food stores, most pet foods are made from the leftovers of chickens, cows, pigs, fish,-which are not fit or cannot be used for human consumption, the nasty smelling hard nuggets, known as Dry pet food is coated with freeze dried grease to bind the stuff & hold it all together, much of this grease is used restaurant grease used in the kitchens & due to be discarded, this is fact, pet food manufacturers buy it by the drum for next to nothing, all this junk food de vitalizes animals & makes them prone to infections & various other maladies for the simple reason there is not enough nutrients in these mass produced dead foods to boost their Immune system & stave off disease & infections. I have 2 Siamese Toms (neutered),they are now 4 years old, they have never needed veterinary services, never been Vaccinated,(you will find that catteries or kennels will not accept cats or dogs for boarding unless they are vaccinated even if you agree to sign a waiver accepting all responsibility for any ailment contracted by your pets during their stay there, if you ask the proprietors for a specific reason they just say **"Its our policy"** because, they never dare to go against the advice of the animals God "The Vet") never had any ailments except Cat flu, at 6 months old which they got over in a week without any inoculations with the help of their own Immune system, They eat mainly raw meat & chicken +lambs or chicken s liver also raw chicken bones & legs also tuna &other raw fish, their coat is sleek & their blue eyes bright, they hunt, fight & sleep & play like any cat should, all on natural raw food, they are not house cats either, they have the run of the house & also all the areas & gardens around the house, including the neighbours & the neighbours cats also whose food they sometimes steal as all cats do, try this regime for your pet, its natural & you know what they are eating., It is also interesting to note that animals in the wild rarely, if ever, have any incidence of cancer or the common diseases normally associated with domestic pets, experts contend that this is because of their diet which is a combination of raw plants & fruits & raw meat (other animals they have killed).

In 1942 Dr. Francis Pottenger Jnr.MD.F.A.C.P. conducted a 10year experiment with hundreds of cats after he ran out of cooked pet food due to the high number of cats being donated to his research lab. where he conducted research into feline diseases, in desperation he got raw meat & organs also bones from a local meat plant which he fed to a number of cats, he noticed they liked this new diet & began to thrive on it, as he continued to feed them this raw meat & raw milk diet, the cats being fed the cooked food & some commercial pet food looked dull & lethargic in comparison also they were more prone to infections & bone diseases & other conditions peculiar to cats, kittens which were fed cooked foods were more prone to skeletal deformities particularly skull deformities, the cats fed on raw meats, fish & veg.& cod liver oil progressed by leaps & bounds, he was so impressed he put his findings into book form & it has become a standard scientific reference work, the book is **"Pottengers cats, a study in nutrition"** by Dr.Francis Pottenger jnr. MD.F.A.C.P.

See also the numerous articles on pets & pet care in "Shirley's Wellness Café" on the internet.

CHAPTER 18

NATURES REMEDIES
PLANTS, TREES, FRUITS & HERBS

GOD in his wisdom has provided remedies in nature to heal or prevent the diseases & disorders we are prone to in our modern society, These remedies have been around for thousands of years but the failure of many modern medicines to treat our illnesses effectively, not to mention the numerous side effects, has created a revival of Herbal Medicine.However, this does NOT mean you should bin all your Prescription Medicines & convert to Herbal remedies immediately, this is Dangerous to say the least & also irresponsible, The proper way is to gradually reduce your Proscription medication & at the same time replace it with the appropriate Herbal equivalent partly to counteract the side effects of the reduced medication & partly to build up your bodies systems in preparation for the time when you are Drug free.

Listed below are selected common diseases, some major, some minor, but all treatable with herbal treatments & with little no side effects,

Note also that herbal or metabolic remedies usually take a lot longer to take effect, some take longer than others but get there eventually, its just a matter of patience so don't expect results overnight.

ANGINA
BROMELAINE (raw pineapple enzyme)
L.CARNITINE (oxygen enhancer)
CO.ENZYME Q10 (reduces chest pains)

HEART DISEASE
GARLIC & ONION (lowers cholesterol)
VITAMIN E (inhibits cholesterol)
VITAMIN B6 (deficiency of B6 major cause of heart disease)
MAGNESIUM (deficiency linked with heart disease, sudden cardiac death, heart attacks, irregular heart rhythms)
BROMELAINE (anti-inflammatory, inhibits platelet accumulation)
GINKO BILOBA (antioxidant, enhances heart efficiency, improves blood vessel elasticity)
HAWTHORN (dilates coronary arteries, decreases lactic acid)
GINGER (lowers cholesterol)
BILBERRY (decreases inflammation, strengthens artery walls)
POMOGRANATE (good all round fruit, very potent anti oxidant, good for heart conditions) The juice is 3 times more potent than Green Tea or Red Wine & also contains vitamins A,C,E, & Iron.

CARDIAC ARRYTHMIAS
Supplements to help maintain a steady heartbeat & Rhythm, Calcium Chelate+ magnesium (helps

maintain regular heartbeat & helps muscle repair) Coenzyme Q10 (general heart tonic) L. Carnitine (reduces Triglycerides) Selenium+ Vitamin E (powerful antioxidants) Vitamin E (thins blood naturally) Potassium (essential for electrolyte balance) Fish Oil (heart tonic)

HERBAL REMEDIES
KAVA –KAVA (eases Anxiety)
VALERIAN (helps sleep)
CAMOMILE (relaxant, similar to Kava-Kava)
HAWTHORN (Cardiovascular herb, reduces blood pressure, strengthens heart muscle)

HIGH BLOOD PRESSURE
HAWTHORN (lowers blood pressure by relaxing & dilating artery walls, used as a treatment for Congestive heart failure, Irregular heartbeats & Angina)
GARLIC (lowers blood pressure & cholesterol,)
COLEUS (FORSKOLIN) used in India to treat high blood pressure & Asthma.
DANDELION (increases urine flow without loss of Potassium)

HIGH CHOLESTROL
VITAMIN B3 (lowers total cholesterol)

GUGGUL (from myrrh tree) Gugulipid protects heart from free radical damage, helps lower cholesterol.

ARTICHOKE (blocks absorption of cholesterol ,inhibits cholesterol production in Liver)

PSYLLIUM (the seeds reduce high cholesterol & triglyceride levels)

GARLIC (helps lower cholesterol)

OSTEOPOROSIS

STINGING NETTLE (natures multivitamin pill) contains Iron, Calcium, Magnesium ,Phosphorus,& Protein.

HORSETAIL (diuretic, also is a major source of Silica, which helps strengthen bones, nails & hair.)

RED CLOVER (contains Isoflavones which act as a mild form of Oestrogen)

ALFALFA(general vitality builder)

SIBERIAN GENSING (general tonic & overall health booster, helps body adapt to increased workload& helps increase alertness)

COLDS & FLU

ECHINACEA (stimulates white cell activity & boosts immune system)

LICQUORICE (stimulates immune cell production & interferon production, is also an Anti-inflammatory)

ELDER (the trees berries are good flu fighters, contains compounds that inhibit flu virus enzyme)

GARLIC (inhibits or kills broad range of microbes ,active against cold & flu viruses)

DEPRESSION

ST. JOHNS WORT (mood lifter)

OATS (strong medicinal qualities for depression, anxiety & stress (dried oat seeds)

LAVENDER (relaxing antidepressant, also promotes sleep)

GINKO BILOBA (increases blood flow, soothes nervous system)

KAVA KAVA (alleviates anxiety states & depression)

DIABETES

GYMNEMA Gymnemic acid blocks tongues ability to sense sweetness (only when the herb is placed on tongue) Gymnema also appears to stimulate Pancreas to produce more insulin & enhances activity of insulin ,helpful in type 1 &

2 diabetes.

FENUGREEK The seeds lower blood glucose& insulin levels Cholesterol & Triglycerides while increasing HDL(good cholesterol) Seeds also contain 50%fibre which slows down the stomachs emptying time & delays absorption of glucose from small intestine, resulting in lower blood sugar.

BILBERRYContainsAnthocyanidins & Proanthocyanidins (types of flavinoids) & have a beneficial effect on capillaries& helps avoid damage to these, thus reducing many diabetic complications.

GRAPESEED (has identical qualities of Bilberry)

FATIGUE

SIBERIAN GINSING (much favoured fatigue buster, safe for long term use)

PANAX GINSING (similar to Siberian Ginsing but is milder& less stimulating) **p/s not advisable for anyone with high blood pressure.**

LIQUORICE (adrenal tonic, also has Anti-viral & Anti-inflammatory properties) Contra- indicated for people with High blood pressure, Heart or

Liver disease or diabetes)
REISHI (increases energy, supports immune system, calms & also improves sleep)
ASTRAGALUS (strengthens immune system, good for digestion & lung function, pleasant taste)
PEPPERMINT (mildly stimulating, eases tension & anxiety& gastro-intestinal upsets, drink as a tea)
ROSEMARY (gentle Stimulant for nervous & circulatory systems, helps lift depression,& may improve memory.)

ARTHRITIS
CAPSICUM (strong analgesic & anti-inflamatory)
EVENING PRIMROSE (very effective anti-inflamatory ,especially in Rhumatoid Arthritis)
STINGING NETTLE (recommended because of high Boron
Content(,steam the leaves to remove sting)
GINGER Used a lot in India for Arthritis, Gingerol inhibits production of Prostaglandins(involved in inflammation),can be very effective.
GREEN TEA (contains Polyphenols ,pure green

tea is widely used in China ,helps relieve symptoms of Arthritis)

TUMERIC (inhibits production of Prostaglandins ,can also be applied to the joint as a poultice for pain relief)

YUCCA (extract of Yucca reduces Pain, Swelling & Stiffness)

WILLOW (contains Salicylic Acid, a chemical found in Aspirin, good for pain)

PINEAPPLE (Raw pineapple contains Bromelaine ,a good anti-inflammatory).

As you can imagine it would require a book to document all the ailments that Herbs & Fruits are used to treat, these are just a few to give you an idea of the broad spectrum of conditions that these Alternative treatments are used for, these remedies have been used for Centuries in the Far east & the Middle east as well as Russia & Scandinavian countries, many of these countries use these preparations in conjunction with modern medicine or on their own & find them very effective.

CHAPTER 19

THE DANGERS OF WHITE SUGAR

There are hardly any edible foods on supermarket shelves that do not contain sugar in some form, almost all manufactured foods contain sugar, some more than others, manufacturers who have been told by the government watchdog to reduce the sugar content in certain products get around this legislation by subtle labelling, they call sugar by other names to confuse the issue so that when the sugar conscious shopper reads the label to check the ingredients they will not notice that the sugar content has not really been reduced very much, if at all, because it is now disguised & listed as other ingredients, but in reality these are just other names for good old Sugar, Carbohydrate is a favourite label by which sugar is disguised, this label covers a multitude of sins, Carbohydrate is a term which describes a compound comprising

Carbon, Hydrogen, & Oxygen, Sugar can be grouped with other Carbohydrates also, increasing the number of ways it can be disguised.

Refined sugar is called **SUCROSE,** this is the stuff you put in your Tea & Coffee, its also present in Soft drinks, Sodas, Cakes, Ice cream, Cereals, etc…..Refined sugar is manufactured from cane & beet extract, it has its Salts ,Fibres, Proteins, Vitamins & Minerals removed to leave a white Crystalline substance totally bereft of any nutritional content.

Sugars contained in natural whole foods are easily metabolized by the body, **FRUCTOSE,** (found in fruits), has the necessary Vitamins & Minerals to convert into **GLUCOSE** (blood sugar),necessary for energy, Sucrose, being devoid of these essential nutrients cannot metabolize fully in our bodies, thus giving rise to Metabolites such as PYRUVIC ACID & other abnormal, unstable sugars.

These toxic by- products interfere with cell respiration thus affecting our breathing to a certain extent, these rogue, toxic metabolites are known as Free Radicals. (These are the body's Terrorists)

Doctor Joseph Mercola after much research stated(27/08/2000) "Another reason to avoid sugar is to slow down the ageing process, if you want to stay looking young, it is important to limit sugar to the smallest possible amount, it is the most significant factor that accelerates ageing".

"Refined sugar can cause **Copper deficiency,** which reduces the elasticity of veins & arteries, leading to Aneurism & Stroke" (M.Fields..Journal of Clinical Nutrition..1983)

Excess Sucrose toxins accumulate in the bloodstream in the form of Fatty Acids & are stored as excess fat in the inactive areas of the body... e.g. **Belly, Thighs, Hips, Breasts**,& **Triceps** (back of upper arm).

Sucrose also impairs the functioning of vital organs causing a hormonal imbalance, creating **Lethargy, Abnormal Blood pressure, Depletion of Vitamin C reserves** threatening the Cardiovascular system, **Mineral depletion** is also a cause of **A.D.D.& A.D.H.D.** in children, it impairs brain function leading to **Increased emotional instability, Concentration difficulties, Hyperactivity & Violence** both in the classroom

& at home.

It is a well proven fact that many children with A.D.D. or A.D.H.D have made quite amazing recoveries from these illnesses just by cutting out all refined sugars, Stimulants, Artificial preservatives & Colorants, many of them done this by cutting out most or all Cereals,& especially Fizzy drinks & concentrating on more fresh fruit (not canned, canned fruit is full of sweeteners) & veg.+real fruit juice (not from concentrate) to further stabilize them they were also taken off ALL medication (most of them Psychiatric drugs)

Refined sugar is also a significant factor in Type 2 Diabetes.

CHAPTER 20 (A)

SACCHARIN (known as "The Pink" because of its wrapper)

Saccharin has been around for a long time as a substitute for sugar but Saccharin has problems of its own, in its pure state saccharin is 500 times as sweet as sugar cane, the commercial grade sold over the counter is 350 times as sweet, This is also categorized as Carbohydrate.

More sinister is the fact that after tests in Canada in 1977 it was officially termed a **CARCINOGEN**,(a cancer causing agent) The American government was about to ban it but such was its popularity among slimmers, millions of them bought all the stocks up, Congress then ,in response to this let it stay on the market with a health warning, but the U.S. Toxicology dept. still put it on its Carcinogen list. It still remains controversial & caution is advised.(15)

The best alternative is pure Unrefined Brown sugar if a sweetener is required, this is pure cane sugar with all the proteins, minerals & vitamins intact, or another alternative is Blackstrap Molasses, which also has all the nutrients, maybe not as small or convenient to carry around but an awful lot safer.

CHAPTER 20 (B)

ASPARTAME (known as "The Blue" because of its wrapper)

Aspartame, like its buddy Saccharin is also small & handy to carry around, but it also is very controversial, you have seen it under the brand names **Splenda, NutraSweet, Equal Spoonful, Equal Measure,** it is also found in many soft drinks, especially Carbonated[fizzy] drinks There was growing concern over its Neurological effects as far back as 1974 & its approval was blocked by Neuroscientist Dr. John.w.Olney on the basis of research he done, The manufacturer G.D.Searle,s research practices were also suspect, but approval was granted in 1983 for production.

In 1985 G.D.Searle was bought by Monsanto & Searle Pharmaceuticals & NutraSweet became separate corporate businesses.

Researcher Alex Constantine said in his essay

"Sweet Poison" that Aspartame may account for up to **75%** of the adverse food reactions reported to the American F.D.A., due primarily to its ability to affect Neurological processes in humans.(many M.S. sufferers have noticed a vast overall improvement in their condition since eliminating drinks & foods with Aspartame in them) Some conditions with Side effects & contributing factors that have been attributed to Aspartame are,. **M.S, Alzheimer's disease, A.L.S, Memory loss, Hormonal problems, Hearing loss, Epilepsy, Parkinson's disease, A.I.D.S, Dementia, Brain lesions & Neuroendocrine disorders,** Risks to Children, Infants & Pregnant women are also noted.

DR. Joseph Mercola said, "It is the only Chemical Warfare weapon available in mass quantities on the grocery counter & promoted in the media".

So the message is Avoid fizzy drinks like the plague, also drinks made from concentrate, Read the label & if Aspartame is among the ingredients, forget it & if you want to live longer & remain "With It", don't use Aspartame as a sweetener in tea or anything else.

CHAPTER 21

THE AMAZING BENEFITS OF FISH OIL

Doctor Dave Woynarowski M.D. done an exhaustive study of the benefits of fish oil, this is a brief summary of his findings…………..

1. Fish oil prevents second heart attacks better than any drug it was tested against.

2. Fish oil is probably the best "medicine" available to prevent sudden Cardiac death.

3 Fish oil makes Asprin's "blood thinning benefits pale into insignificance, also those who cannot tolerate Asprin will have no problem with the taste of pharmaceutical grade fish oil, as opposed to normal fish oil bought in stores.

4. Fish oil has been used effectively in the treatment of Alzheimers Disease.

5. Fish oil improves memory, I.Q.& helps obliterate age related Memory lapses.

6. Fish oil plays a key role in brain development, in a Scottish study of young children, fish oil improved cognitive & visual skills,- making them smarter than kids who did not use it.

7. Fish oil helps people with M.S.

8. Fish oil lowers blood pressure [this is a widely tested fact]

9. Fish oil reduces the incidence of Stroke caused by the clotting of Brain blood vessels.

10 Fish oil lowers Triglicerides & raises good H.D.L.cholesterol ,reducing the risk of heart disease.

11. Fish oil is a very potent antioxidant & one of the few that cross the blood brain barrier. I call it the ultimate antioxidant & in many cases the only one you may need.

12 Fish oil improves personality, mood & mental disorders.

13. Fish oil is a potent natural anti-depressant !

14. Fish oil improves the health of cartilage & joints!

15. Fish oil improves the ratio of Testosterone to its metabolite, D.H.T., & in studies was shown to be useful in treating Prostate, Colon, & Breast Cancers.

16. Fish oil simultaneously improves hormone levels & improves the health of joints, thus making it the perfect anti-ageing supplement as well as a superb supplement for Athletes, speeding recovery time from hard workouts.!

17 Fish oil balances hormone levels in the body, thus having many benefits,one of which is sounder, deeper sleep so that you wake up refreshed & invigorated.

18. Fish oil reduces inflammation in the lungs & can be used to treat Allergies Asthma & Eczema.

When you look at the benefits of Fish oil, & this is only a fraction of the multitude of Natural remedies made available to us by the Creator God himself, its not hard to imagine how easy it could be to get healthy & stay healthy & at the same time save a fortune in medical bills Thoroughbred animals are fed the best nutrients & animal feed money can buy to keep them in pristine condition how much more valuable are our own bodies, do we treat them as well as we treat our animals judging by the multitude of ailments we suffer, I don't think we do, Get a life! In the words of a famous song, "Get on your feet, get out & make it happen".,NOW.!!!

CHAPTER 22

PHYSICAL FITNESS

Physical fitness is a subject not spoken of very often in scripture, the reason for this is not very apparent, even though the Greeks were fitness fanatics, even to the extent of instituting the first Olympiad, but it is a subject that is of paramount importance to maintaining physical & spiritual wellbeing, A physical derclict is not a good advertisement for the saving & keeping power of God, God saves you to serve him, but you cannot serve him,(or your family) effectively if you are physically ill because of self neglect, this is **NOT** the Devil making you ill, It is yourself making you ill because of a combination of **laziness, lack of self discipline, inattention to proper diet, & generally letting yourself go to the dogs,** for whatever reason.

When you are physically unfit it does not help your spiritual walk with God because being unfit will make you more prone to physical ailments & this in turn will occupy your mind & detract from your spiritual walk.

The Apostle Paul said "Bodily exercise profiteth little", or as the margin of the King James translation says, "It profits for a little while"(1st. Timothy 4-8) I believe this was Pauls own opinion & not necessarily an inspired statement of fact, because it is an established scientific fact that bodily exercise profits a lot, physical fitness contributes a lot to the general health & wellbeing of a person ,& the effects can be life long, & not only contribute to a long life but also a more productive & meaningful life, you cannot serve God to your full capacity if you are incapacitated because of illness due to self neglect, Alas, being healthy does not come automatically, even to Gods people, you have to work at it, & once you have got it you have to keep working at it to maintain it, being healthy is not just a matter of eating the proper foods, its also a matter of keeping your body in good shape by exercising & toning the joints & muscles, this not only helps to prevent Arthritis & other related conditions but also prevents the muscles atrophying (wasting away) from lack of use, Exercise also stimulates the heart to beat faster & pump blood around the body faster to supply the individual muscles & tissues that are working overtime, all this activity requires more nutrients to nourish & rejuvenate the cells & supply building material for more muscle, & to maintain the health of the bones & tissues, blood is manufactured primarily in the long bones & stored in the Spleen & various other organs, this is why your body needs to be constantly fed with the best nutrients to maintain optimum health, but its no good consuming the best nutrients if your muscles are wasting away & your joints are creaking & groaning in protest because of your inactivity, this is when your ailments begin,& it can be a long & sometimes painful road to full recovery, which is why a proper all round fitness regime is a must, not just walking a couple of miles a day, or doing a few sit ups or a few press ups, fitness is beneficial for all ages & all conditions, the fitter you are the faster you will recover from injury, or an operation & if you are unfortunate enough to contract a disease, provided your immune system is intact & functioning well you should be able to mount a major assault on that disease or foreign body & your physical fitness will play a major role in the process,. PS.-As you get older your Immune system begins to deteriorate, therefore it is essential to keep it boosted & fuelled with adequate vitamins to maintain its integrity & effectiveness, I have no doubt that the patriarchs & indeed the new testament saints were reasonably fit considering they had to do a lot of manual work in connection with their everyday professions, Many of the patriarchs were Landowners, farmers or Shepherds of sorts & were probably involved in the day to day running of their estates, Peter & some of the early Disciples were Fishermen which would entail a lot of physical energy & strength to handle the boats & also the nets, especially if they were full of fish, Paul also was self employed as a Tent maker, I would assume the tents in those regions would be the Arab type tent so common in the middle east even today, even with an assistant, it would entail a lot of heavy work folding & pulling into shape the tent materials, & what of our Lord, Jesus himself helped his Father in his Carpenters workshop, which entailed a lot of heavy work, the wood would have been of various sizes & carried I would assume either manually or on a cart or donkey from the forest or wherever it was obtained then sawed manually & planed & finished manually, hard work especially if the wood was cedar or oak, People have often assumed Jesus was a fairly muscular man because of his work with his father(Joseph) & not at all the thin, wimpish figure that he is commonly portrayed as being, but in the interests of historical accuracy there is ample evidence that Jesus spent a lot of his time from his teenage years until he was 30 in & around Britain travelling with his uncle Joseph of Armithea on his frequent business trips, Joseph was a Tin merchant & also owned tin mines in Britain as well as being an influential member of the Sanhedrin like Nicodemas.(16)

Physical fitness is not just beneficial for you, you have to think of your family, especially if they are young, being fit means you can play with them, keep up with them, be competitive with them, participate in their sports, their games, you being fit means a lot to them, because you can relate to them better, communicate better,& understand them & their needs better, it means they don't see you as a broken down old wreck, out of touch with them & their needs, but rather a responsible parent who is interested enough in the welfare & wellbeing of their family to make the effort to be on a fitness level where they can participate in their children's various activities & be an active member of the family "team", to be a participant, not a spectator, wether we like to believe it or not, children want their parents to be role models, they want to look up to them, to believe in them,& if they don't get leadership & guidance & a desirable role model to follow in their parents, they will turn to other sources for a role model & guidance,& in many cases emulate their lifestyle, its your responsibility & your duty to God & to your family to ensure this does not happen, you can certainly pray about it & this is commendable, but it will not make you fit or healthy, praying is not enough, you have to act, get off your butt & do whatever it takes to get fit & healthy & when you get to where you want to be, do whatever it takes to stay there, believe me, your family will respect you for it &God will bless you for it.

CHAPTER 23

STRESS!!! A COMMON KILLER

The causes of stress are many & varied & so are the physical & mental illnesses attributed to this condition, when you are stressed your body produces excess amounts of **Adrenalin& Noradrenalin** to prepare your body for what it perceives is an emergency situation, this sudden rush of these **"emergency** "chemicals gets your body into top gear very quickly to facilitate a quick response to the situation (these are known as the" "Fight or Flight" chemicals), this may be a handy response to have in some situations, but certainly not all the time, because there is a down side to all this, viz.—other chemicals are also at work in times of stress triggered by the same old Stress hormones, Cortisol is one of these, Cortisol releases fat & sugar into your system at this time (but also reduces the efficiency of your immune system)

All these changes make it easier for you to Fight or run away, unfortunately these chemical changes are less helpful if you are not in a position to utilize them, it can be a nightmare if you are stressed out on eg.-a train, bus, aircraft, office, or a car(possibly one of the causes of Road Rage)ect.---where you cannot vent, or release your stress in some way, over time these chemical changes that are produced in your body can damage your physical & mental health, unless the symptoms are detected early & the situation rectified before it gets out of hand.

Stress comes about when you are not in control of a given situation & more times than not you are not in control because of the way you feel, the way you feel could be Psychological, but more often than not it is physical, your body is responding to the way you have treated it by producing pain or severe discomfort to alert you to its plight & warn you of impending danger if you don't do something soon to alleviate the situation.

People who eat healthy & are fit usually feel good & look good, this contributes considerably to a positive attitude which in turn has an influence on the bodys hormones to strengthen the immune system & promote cell growth as well as accelerating the healing process of injuries or post operative recuperation & assists in the elimination of "**Free radicals**".(no, this is not a left wing political party)

Although most, if not all diseases or disorders are associated with, or caused by, poor nutrition, STRESS is also a major causative factor in many disorders & must be considered as a major factor in exacerbating & accelerating the destructive course many diseases take, the following is a short summary of Stress related disorders,

DISORDERS OF THE DIGESTIVE SYSTEM
A ….Ulcers of the stomach & intestines.
B….Ulcerative colitis.

C...Loss of appetite
D...Hiccups.
E...Irritable bowel syndrome.
F...Swallowing difficulties.

CIRCULATORY SYSTEM
A...High blood pressure.
B...Abnormal heartbeats [premature ventricular contractions, paroximal tachycardia ,ect.--]
C...Angina pectoris.
D...Heart attacks[sudden death & myocardial infarction]
E...Strokes

GENITO-URINARY SYSTEM.
A... Lack of menstruation.
B...Vaginismus.
C..Frequent or painful urination.
D...Impotence.
E.. Dysfunctional uterine bleeding.
F..False pregnancy.
G..Infertility.

NERVOUS SYSTEM.
A...Headaches of most types.
B...Epilepsy.
C...Panic attacks.

D...Tremors.

E...Suicide.

GLANDULAR DISORDERS

A...Thyroid disorders.

B...Diabetes[types I & 2 affecting both the onset & course]

C...Chronic pancreatitis.

ALLERGIC & IMMUNOLOGIC DISORDERS.

A...Chronic fatigue syndrome.

B...Hives.

C....Hay fever

D...Asthma attacks.

E...Poor vaccine response.

The solution to all this self inflicted misery is to return to a proper, wholesome, Bible based dietary regime which must, as a prerequisite include a thorough detox programme to eliminate the free radicals & other cell destroying junk from your system & pave the way for the regeneration process which will be achieved through proper nutrition combined with selective metabolic therapy.

CHAPTER 24

FEAR & WORRY

A famous American Pastor back in the 50.s once stated.—"Worry is a mild form of Atheism", Doubt & unbelief reflects on our faith, or lack of faith, in God, & contributes greatly to our bodies decline into chaos, If we already have a physical ailment Fear & worry activate mechanisms in the brain which in turn constrict the blood vessels (this is part of the fight or flight response we discussed in the last chapter) if this condition lasts long enough it can cause a lot of damage to organs & tissues through a reduced blood supply, this also slows or even stops wound healing,& as more cells die Sickness & disease follow, & eventually Death, You can actually worry yourself into the grave.

"The fear of man bringeth a snare"(Proverbs 29-25) The fear of what man can do to us can snare us & cause anxiety & worry, this then can lead to the domino effect mentioned above, The fear of man can lead to Misery, Resentfulness, Tension, both in the workplace & at home, it can get so bad that we even contemplate Suicide as a way of escape, I really hate fear, Its destructive, physically & mentally, its an awful thing to live in fear, In my experience as a Psychiatric nurse I saw the manifestations of fear many times, in the form of Schizophrenia, Reactive & Endogenous depression, Manic depression, Alcoholic withdrawal symptoms(D.T.s) also many other disorders too numerous to mention here which generated Fear, Worry,& Anxiety states leading to sickness & dietary problems.

Some of the Physical problems associated with stress & anxiety are listed here.

MUSCLE & JOINT DISORDERS.
A...Low back syndrome.
B...Neck spasms.
C...Rheumatoid arthritis.
D...Myasthenia gravis.

INFECTIONS.
A...Common cold.
B...Infectious mononucleosis.

C...Chronic tuberculosis.
D...Strep throat.

INFLAMMATORY & SKIN DISEASES
A...Neurodermatitis.
B...Reynauds disease.
C...Systemic lupus erythematosus.

NUTRITIONAL & DRUG DISORDERS
A...Anorexia nervosa.
B...Obesity.
C...Drug addictions[cocaine ,alcohol, nicotine, caffeine,]
D...Vitamin toxicity.

CANCERS.
A...Lung cancer
B...Gastric cancer.
C...Childhood cancers.
D...Breast cancer.
E...Numerous other types.

Stress comes about when we forget to include God in our everyday lives, the words of a very famous hymn are very appropriate.

O What peace we often forfeit

O what needless pain we bear

All because we do not carry

Every thing to God in prayer

"But they that wait upon the lord shall renew their strength, they shall mount up with wings as eagles, they shall run & not be weary & they shall walk & not faint".(Isaiah 40-31)

t The Bibles answer to STRESS is peace with God through Jesus Christ, the presence of the Holy Spirit in a persons life dispels Fear & Anxiety, the twin evils that contribute to stress.

John the Apostle stated it perfectly in Ist. John 4-18 "There is no fear in love, but perfect love casteth out all fear, because fear hath torment, he that feareth is not made perfect in love,"

Luke the Physician in Luke 21 v-25-26 gives a scenario of the end times & gives a Prophetic account of real fear,eg.—"And there shall be signs in the sun & in the moon & in the stars,& upon the earth, **DISTRESS OF NATIONS WITH PERPLEXITY,** the sea & the waves roaring".(People in turmoil)**"MENS HEARTS**

FAILING THEM FOR FEAR, & looking after those things which are coming on the earth, for the powers of the heavens shall be shaken."Peace with God is the only answer we have to the plague of fear, get it & lose your fear.

CHAPTER. 25

THE DEMON DRINK

SOLOMON got it right when he said in the book of Proverbs,.."Wine is a mocker, Strong drink is raging, and whosoever is deceived thereby is not wise"(proverbs,20:1)

"Who hath woe ?Who hath sorrow ?

Who hath contentions ? Who hath babblings ?

Who hath wounds without cause ? Who hath redness of eyes ?They that tarry long at the wine, they that go to seek mixed wine!

Look not thou upon the wine when it is red,When it giveth his colour in the cup, when it moveth itself aright.

At the last it biteth like a serpent, and stingeth like an Adder".(proverbs ch.23-.v.29-32)

This is the true picture of the rewards of Alcohol, the picture you will never see on the advertisement billboards or in the glossy magazine ads.

The booze manufacturers will not touch on the subject of "Alcopops"or Shandy,s, designed to get the younger age groups hooked on the taste of booze legally, in preparation for the real thing when they are older, although in most cases many under age drinkers usually get the real stuff by one means or another, nowadays its not unusual for pre teens to be found drunk, and usually at all hours of the morning, Where are their parents at this time? certainly not watching out for them, that's for sure! In many cases they are probably as drunk as their kids, & probably don't even know what day it is, never mind where their kids are.

What an environment to rear children in.

Space would not permit me to mention the countless homes & marriages that have been wrecked by boozed up partners or the numerous careers that have been scuppered by drink sodden aspiring executives who started out drinking socially to be accepted in the business circles & ended up being drunk as a skunk more often than they were sober & just as smelly, or the Business man who established a thriving business & then drunk his profits until the business went down the tubes, I fully accept all drinkers are certainly not Alcoholics & many can drink moderately & still maintain a good marriage & a business, but the potential is ever present to over indulge & let the booze take control especially if stress or distress is a factor & Alcohol is to hand,. This is when life changing events can so very easily happen, very fast.

The driver who is over the limit or even the driver who has only had a few beers, thinks he /she is capable because their sense of reason is up the left & so is their judgment, & very often tragedy is not far away.Indeed many newspapers carry accounts of drunk drivers so drunk they drove on the wrong side of the road into oncoming traffic, or others who run someone down but were too drunk to even notice the body being tossed over the bonnet from the impact, or in more recent years the carnage of cars full of young people, most of them dead or badly injured as the car was wrapped around a tree after hitting it at high speed as it spun out of control due to the driver being drunk & incapable of controlling it, These drivers don't only kill themselves but usually all or most of those in the car also, When these demon drivers get behind the wheel, all reason & intelligence goes out the window as the demon drink numbs their brain, There are also many recent accounts of young people falling over hotel balconies to their death, or serious injury while on holiday, or others who have drowned, having fallen into the hotel pool & being too drunk to save themselves,(holiday or travel insurance companies will not cover these type of accidents if drink is involved,)There is also the numerous cases of spiked drinks or girls just too drunk to know what is happening, until someone tells them the next day, but as if this was not enough, many Pubs & clubs are open till 1am or 2am.& the news is full of reports of an increase in the number of drink fuelled fights & brawls, sometimes even murders, & the Politicians who pass the licensing laws extending the Pub & Club drinking hours say its good for the economy & the public demand ,What can you do with Government Ministers like that ?

The brain has a protective system to prevent toxins from getting to the brain cells, its called the Blood Brain Barrier, unfortunately this barrier cannot prevent the toxins of Alcohol getting across & when it does it wrecks havoc.It attacks the centres in the brain that control Inhibitions, Memory, Speech, Reason, Morals, as well as Movement coordination, & muscle coordination, this is why many people with hangovers the next day cannot remember what happened, or why they were incontinent, or indeed why they done the things they did ,or said the things they said.

Alas this sad tale of woe is not the end, not by a long shot, in addition to the list above the SHORT TERM effects of regular Alcohol consumption are:-
The Central Nervous System is depressed
Judgment & Memory are affected, Perception, Drowsiness & poor sleep patterns are also affected.

LONG TERM side effects are,--
Pancreatic disorders (pancreatitis)

Heart problems.(atrial fibrillation, can be common in binge drinkers especially young people, also Cardiomyopathy)
High blood pressure problems
Irritation of the Stomach & Small intestine.
Elimination of B cells

In severe cases especially the consumption of Spirits, liver Damage is a very real probability, The Liver is the Laboratory of the body, the blood flows through it & is filtered, all the toxins & other foreign bodies harmful to the body are shunted out via the numerous outlets in the body, but if the Liver is damaged its ability to function at maximum capacity is severely limited, in more severe cases the Liver is so badly necrosed (scarred & withered) & the blood flow through it so badly restricted, the poisonous substances so easily filtered out in a healthy liver, spread into other organs via the blood, & contaminate the body, This is **CIRROSIS** a deadly disease & incurable without a transplant, by the time the liver is in this state the man/woman is already an ALCOHOLIC, & Doctors are reluctant to transplant a liver into this type of person, they don't think they are worthy of it.

By the time people get to this stage in their drinking career they are virtually Human Derelicts, reduced to the dregs of society, so low they could walk under a snakes belly with a top hat on, sounds funny but its true, Alcohol can reduce you to this, the Bible states "Wherefore let him that thinketh he stand take heed lest he fall" (1st. Corinthians.ch.10v.12) Wise words indeed.

Unless you have lived in a cave all your days I am quite sure you are very familiar with all this, The hardened drinker as well as the mildest teetotal has heard it all before & indeed many know from bitter experience,

THAT IS THE BAD NEWS

THIS IS THE GOOD NEWS.....YOU CAN BE DELIVERED!!!

YOU CAN BE FREE FROM THE DEMON "DRINK" !!!

Turning over a new leaf is good ,....but alas, not good enough.
Transforming your home is good ....but not good

enough.

Transforming your lifestyle is good too….but still not good enough.

Going to live on a desert island may help,….but its not a lasting solution.

Going to church would definitely help…but would not be enough.

Drugs or rehab clinics may help in the short term…but again, these are not the answer.

There is only **ONE** way you can beat your demons & its not with A.A.or any similar organization, excellent & helpful though these may be, you do not need renewal, you need **REGENERATION**, A total overhaul from the inside out, you need your life turned around, nothing or nobody on this earth is capable of doing this, except the one who created life, GOD himself, he knows you & your body better than anyone & he knows what you need, you need a Regeneration of Mind, Body, & Spirit, brought about by the power that created the universe, the Holy Spirit of God, **This can change your Nature, this can make you a New creation in Jesus Christ**, your Attitude will change, your Values will change, your total Life will change,.for the better, booze will no longer hold any attraction for you, they say once you have been an Alcoholic you are always an Alcoholic, this is certainly true if you are trying to effect a cure in your own strength, & beat the bottle by conventional means, but this is where the similarity ends, when you accept Jesus into your life & he transforms you by the Power of Regeneration, you become a new person, you are cured totally from your Addictions to Alcohol, Drugs, or whatever you need to be cured from, the Demons are gone, you can say with total authority from God himself that you are no longer an addict of any sort, No Doctor, No Clinic, No Treatment regime, No Guru can give you this guarantee, Only GOD himself can, & will, but you have to ask him, & you have to accept his terms, Do this & you can be free from your demons.& be the man/woman you want to be.

CHAPTER. 26

45 FOODS RICH IN VITAMIN B 17

As mentioned in previous chapters Vitamins & Minerals are the essential building blocks of our bodies, the roles they play in maintaining the bodies integrity & assisting in the smooth operation of the numerous systems are many & varied. A key vitamin is B17 (or Latrille as it is sometimes known),this vitamin is not only a Cancer killer it is also a cell rejuvenator, & regular consumption will go a long way to help maintain optimum health.

The following 45 foods are easily obtained & contain various amounts of B17, some more than others, you cannot consume enough of these, indeed the more B17 you consume the less you will need to see your Doctor, because you will be that much more healthier, The following is a list of common fruits & foods containing the Vitamin

B17.

ALFALFA SPROUTS APPLE SEEDS
APRICOT KERNELS (high concentration)
BUCKWHEAT
BAMBOO SHOOTS CASHEWS
BARLEY (high concentration) CASAVA(tapioca)
BEET TOPS CHERRY KERNELS
BITTER ALMOND (high concentration)
CRANBERRY
BLACKBERRY UCALYPTUS LEAVES
BOYSENBERRY CURRENTS
BREWERS YEAST FAVA BEANS
BROWN RICE FLAX SEEDS
GARBANZO BEANS GOOSEBERRY
GREEN PEAS HUCKLEBERRY
KIDNEY BEANS LENTILS
LIMA BEANS LINSEED MEAT
LOGANBERRIES MACADAMIA NUTS
MILLET MILLET SEED
MULBERRY NECTARINE KERNELS
PEACH KERNELS PEAR SEEDS
PECANS PLUM KERNELS
QUINCE RASBERRY
SORGHUM CANE SYRUP SPINACH

SPROUTS (alfalfa, mung bean, lentil, BITTER ALMONDS
Buckwheat, garbanzo)
SQUASH SEEDS STRAWBERRY
WALNUTS WATERCRESS

PS. The reason Doctors will give for recommending **small** dosages of B 17 is the mistaken belief that since B17 has a Cyanide molecule, the more B17 you eat the more Cyanide will build up in your body & create Cyanide poisoning.

First let me say, as I did in chapter 10 that the Cyanide molecule in B17 has to be formed, it is not free floating & it can only be formed in the presence of the enzyme Beta-glucosidase (found only in Cancer cells) so you cannot get an accumulation of Hydrogen Cyanide as some so called "Specialists" claim, There is also an enzyme which all normal cells have called "Rhodanese," Hydrogen Cyanide cannot live in the presence of Rhodanese, so there is no possibility of a Hydrogen Cyanide molecule escaping & running amok among all the good cells, it could never survive to do any damage.

As a matter of interest Vitamin B12 has a fairly high concentration of Cyanide (Cyanocobalimin)

,it is found in Red meat, Dairy products, & Eggs, it plays a major role in the formation of Red blood cells & is also essential for the maintenance of a healthy Nervous system, A deficiency of this Vitamin can be disastrous, Anaemia being just one of the complications.

I wonder why this Vitamin with its high Cyanide content has not been assaulted by the "Experts."

.There are also at least another 10 or so other fruits containing Cyanide.

It is interesting to note that there has NEVER been any record of anyone anywhere ever suffering from Cyanide poisoning as a result of taking too much Vitamin B17.

Is that not amazing? The truth of the matter is that the "Experts" know all about B17& its mode of operation very well but they don't want you to know, or at least they don't want you to know just how effective it is, so they do what they do best, they try to discredit it.

CHAPTER 27

EIGHT OF THE MOST POTENT IMMUNE SYSTEM BOOSTERS, ALSO VERY HIGH IN ANTI-OXIDANTS, NATURES OWN ANTI-BIOTICS.

1...BROCCOLI

2...BLUEBERRIES / BILBERRIES.

3...GROUND FLAXSEED

4...GARLIC

5...GREEN TEA (Sometimes called Gunpowder tea)

6...SALMON

7...SPINACH

8...TOMATOES

CHAPTER 28

DISEASE CONTROL & SANITATION

One of the fundamentals in the control of diseases is ensuring that they do not spread, this can only be achieved by isolation of the individual who has contracted the disease, to ensure that no one else is infected, in Bible times the Israelites were instructed to isolate any person who was known to be infectious in an area outside the camp, well away from the people, until the high priest deemed he was free of the disease, any one who visited him,(usually relatives or priests, or other friends with food ect.) had to be thoroughly washed in running water & their clothes were thoroughly washed in running water, then left out in the sun to dry, this also ensured that the hot sun & Ultra Violet rays helped to kill any remaining germs. They done all this before returning to the camp, this way all disease was kept to the absolute minimum, Although disease from infected food was rare there was no doubt environmental factors which would have contributed to the spread of disease from time to time, But nevertheless Israel was an example to all the Non Israelite nations around them of the wisdom & practicality of Gods natural healthcare system.

Modern scientific research has proved the validity of the Mosaic Hygiene laws & proved once again that we cannot improve on Gods laws, some of which are briefly outlined here.

(1) Any person who has handled or worked with diseased or dead people (or animals) must wash themselves & their clothes in RUNNING water to prevent bacteria attaching themselves to the persons hands or body, bacteria thrive & hatch out on human body heat, but they are flushed away in running water..

(2) If a person had a running sore he was pronounced unclean, so also was anyone who sat on a seat or bed previously occupied by the unclean person, this person was required to wash himself & either burn or wash his clothes in running water & be isolated outside the camp from 1 to 7 days

depending on the level of contamination deemed by the priest. The seat & bed linen & all other possessions of the person with the running sore was either washed or burned, this prevented the spread of bacteria.

(3)If a person was working in the fields & proper toilets were not available he had to carry with him a small shovel to cover up whatever he had to do to prevent the spread of infection, this was very effective.& practical.

The year **1847 in Austria** was a very sad & bleak year, Many women died in childbirth, the mortality rate for mothers & babies was very high in most hospitals, 1 in 6 in fact ,& it was a long time before the situation changed, The main cause of the high death rate was primarily ignorance on the part of the Doctors, & to a lesser extent the midwives, During the autopsies (usually the dead mothers from the maternity ward) which the medical students did with bare hands, one sight was very common,the abdomen & chest cavity of the dead patient was nearly always filled with pus, a sure sign of rife infection, it was called **"Labour Fever"**. These same students & sometimes Doctors would deliver babies or do vaginal examinations with these same filthy, germ laden hands that had been inside the abdomen of an infected corpse just a few minutes earlier in the morgue next door, After a quick rinse of their hands they would dry them on an old rag or their coats, they then proceeded with the morning round, their hands & clothes still smelling of rotting flesh,. They went from patient to patient doing internal examinations or deliveries, usually without washing their hands between each patient,. Just a few minutes earlier their hands had been in Blood, Pus, & Dead bodies,..Sanitation was non existent, Death was usually inevitable for these unfortunate women, because most of them would have been poor, & unable to afford the necessary nutritious foods or indeed even known about them, to boost their Immune system & give them a fighting chance,. These barbaric medical practices were the norm throughout Europe because no one had even heard of Bacteria, deaths were blamed on, Bad air, Atmospheric conditions, Cosmic conditions, you name it they had a name for it, if a Doctor delivered a baby the death rate was 18% If a midwife delivered it the death rate was only 3%,

The reason was Obvious, Doctors do autopsies,. Midwives do not,. The famous physician **Doctor Semmelweis,** finally introduced strict hand washing, The mortality rate fell from 18% to 1% in 3 months, Typically no one listened to him in medical circles & the death rate remained high for a long time outside his hospital in Vienna.

The ancient Egyptians were experts in Embalming, unfortunately the same germs that killed the Pharaohs & their wealthy friends remained in the corpse because of the humid conditions of the body & the tomb, so when the Physician/Embalmer entered the body to retrieve the organs or do an autopsy the lack of proper hygiene procedures manifested themselves in the transference of germs from corpses to patients resulting in the deaths of many patients & probably the Physician himself, and while all this was going on the Bible had already laid down the ground rules for healthy living in these same circumstances(Numbers19-11)**"He that toucheth the dead body of any man shall be unclean seven days"V.12.."He shall purify himself on the third day and on the seventh day shall be clean" V.13.."Whosoever**

toucheth the dead body of any man and purifyeth not himself defileth the Tabernacle of God and that soul shall be cut off from Israel because the water of separation (purification) was not sprinkled (or, he was not properly washed) o**n him and he is unclean"**.(for 7 days)

Hyssop was used as an antiseptic to wash with in addition to running water.(You remember Jesus was offered Hyssop when he was on the cross, Hyssop was not only an Antiseptic, it also had Anesethic properties).

It was not until **1869** that **Joseph Lister** the famous British Surgeon introduced Antiseptics into medicine, (Carbolic acid) Thousands of years after God had instructed the ancient Israelites in these basic techniques.

Once again we discover the Bible is even more up to date than tomorrows newspaper, numerous so called great discoveries of the middle ages & even more recent centuries were in fact mentioned in the Bible in the Old Testament, but many of the eminent scientists not being familiar with the Bible did not know that the Bible had in fact answered their scientific queries, & the fact that their discoveries were nothing new.EG..—In the middle ages many people thought that the Earth was flat, but Isaiah stated "It is he that sitteth upon the CIRCLE of the Earth"(Isa.40-22)

William Harvey discovered the **"Circulation of the blood"** in 1628 & made medical history, but the Bible had already stated this in Leviticus 17-11.."**For the life of the flesh is in the blood".**

These great revelations have been in the Bible for centuries but only in recent years have scientists discovered & proved their accuracy & scientific basis, genuine science does not conflict with the Bible, it proves its accuracy.

CHAPTER. 29

THE DIETARY PROCESS OF WEIGHT REDUCTION

Having went into great detail about the perils of obesity & the short & long term effects of this dangerous condition it would be remiss of me to preach to you about this without giving you the solution to the problem, but before you can even start to think about losing weight & getting into shape you have got to realize & admit to yourself that you do have a problem & that it will take dedication & determination to do whatever has to be done to get to where you want to be,(or need to be) so that you can look in the mirror & say,"I like what I see."

The principle reason people put on weight is because their intake is more than their output, that is to say they eat a lot but do not exercise or do any other kind of activity to burn off the excess calories, so it accumulates on the body in the form of fat(or Adipose tissue to be medically correct) but when you exercise or otherwise burn energy on a reduced intake of calories your body burns up the fat in your tissues to fuel your exercise, this sounds elementary but it is in fact very scientific, but it also requires close scrutiny of what you eat,(and also when you eat it) But this need not be a chore, weight reduction can be pleasant if you approach it in the right way & in the right frame of mind.,This is very important because attitude is everything, if you have a "positive "attitude you can do almost anything, but a "negative "attitude is very destructive, You have no doubt heard the expression, "Three Square Meals a day" this may sound good but in actual fact its not, because The three square meals are usually large amounts of food eaten for Breakfast, Dinner, and Tea, As discussed in chapter 8 this kind of eating puts a massive strain on the digestive system, the normal, proper way to eat is,5 or 6 small meals per day spread throughout the day,8 or9 pm being the time of the last meal, This is very logical & also eliminates those "peckish "periods when most of the damage is done Drinking water or Tea between times helps to increase the "full" feeling also as well as keeping the body hydrated, Speaking of Tea, Green (also known as Gunpowder tea because of its colour) tea is very beneficial, having many virtues, it is not fermented so its medicinal properties are unaltered, Some of the known health conditions where Green tea has been found to be effective eg.-

A---It helps reduce the risk of Cancer.

B---Helps prevent Gingivitis (periodontal disease)

C---Helps reduce high cholesterol.
D---Helps reduce high blood pressure
E—Helps reduce high triglycerides
F---Boosts immune function
G—Assists prostate health

Green tea is bitter but if you really need it sweetened then pure cane sugar (unrefined) is suitable, this sugar retains all the original nutrients, Blackstrap Molasses is also another alternative, Get the tea loose and use a fine sieve & put the sieve over the cup, or teapot, put 2 spoonfuls into the sieve & pour hot water over it up to the brim& let it sit for 5 minutes, alternatively use a coffee percolator or tea bags, Another alternative drink is blueberries liquidized, or pineapple(raw) liquidized, Blueberries are Super immune system boosters.& Pineapples are full of the enzyme **Bromelaine.**(very useful in metabolic therapy, Bromelaine breaks down the protective coating on Cancer cells)

Breakfast is meant to be light,. **not** eggs, sausages, potato bread ect.....followed by cereals, fruit juice, toast,ect. this is a Continental style breakfast & contrary to popular opinion does **not** set you up for the day.(It conflicts with your body's elimination cycle which is still in full swing) see ch.8

A typical breakfast for anyone on a reduction diet or just trying to maintain a healthy weight would be,-.

8 or 9 am......Two slices of toast(not white bread) & some fruit & either Green tea or Earl Grey with 2 spoonfuls of Manuka honey as a nutritious sweetener (see ch.5) or fruit juice (not from concentrate)+2 Cod Liver oil capsules(1200mg.) (see "Benefits of fish oil"ch.21)

11am Some cream crackers (or similar)Fruit juice (not from concentrate)+grapes or some plums.

1.30 or 2 pm. Lunch...2 rounds cheese on toast or cheese or chicken Pannini.+Tea or Juice.

4.30 or 5 pm HighTea.....Medium sized portions of Broccoli &/or Cauliflower +breast or leg of chicken +tea or fruit juice(taken in sips with food, or 20-30 mins. after)

7 or 8pm,...Some Melon slices or Banana or Orange +fruit juice. Or Green tea +2 spoonfulls of Manuka Honey as a sweetner in the tea & also as an anti-bacterial nutrient.

As you can see this is only a rough guide to a daily routine, obviously these foods can be changed to suit you & your individual preferences, you can also have meat,(bloodless if possible, or "Kosher "as the Jewish communities call it or Halal as Muslims call it) Fish (not battered) Eggs, poached or boiled or scrambled if possible instead of fried

There are also multitudes of various Salad dishes or even some Curry dishes (mild) there are medicinal properties in Curry, Chinese foods like Bamboo shoots or Bean sprouts are also good (Bamboo shoots are rich in Vitamin B17).

CHAPTER 30

THEORY & PRACTICE OF DETOXING THE PROS & CONS

The practice of **Detoxing** as a means of cleansing the body systems is nothing new but it does require either supervision or a relatively good knowledge of Nutrition.

Detoxing is not recommended as a means of losing weight because most Detox regimes involve Low calorie & /or Low carbs (carbohydrates) both of which don't work as weight loss regimes for the following reasons..—

1/..Low Calorie diets are basically Starvation diets which actually have the effect of slowing down the bodys metabolism, because the body detects a reduction in calorie intake & compensates by slowing down the fat burning mechanism to conserve energy.

2/ Low Carbs do not work either because they rob the body of energy & frequently give rise to headaches, tiredness & sickness, this is not the result of detoxifying the body but rather a lack of food since detoxing can cause a shortage of vital nutrients & lower immunity.

Some detox regimes require the individual to eliminate Dairy products like Milk, Eggs, Chicken,ect.---These are good sources of Calcium & cutting these out can lead to a Calcium deficiency, which in turn can lead to Osteoporosis & also fractures can be very slow to heal & require other supplements to replace the lost Calcium.

Strictly speaking a specialized Detox dietary regime is not necessary if a good variety of fresh fruit & vegetables & plenty of natural water,(not bottled), filtered if possible, is available, bottled water tends to have additives, also the plastic material the bottles are made from can also leak chemicals, so if you are abroad & have to use bottled water, if the bottle is not glass drink real fruit juice **(not from concentrate)**or if necessary non alcoholic Table Wine, at least you can be reasonably sure the water content is relatively pure.(purer than the local water at least)

The Detoxifying programme most Metabolic Therapy Clinics will put you on initially to cleanse the body systems is usually based on the good old fresh fruit & veg+natural whole Figs, Prunes, Grapes, ect..—basically what you should be eating on a regular basis anyway.

So you see you don't need to spend extra cash on so called "Specialist Detox Programmes"or detox diets if you follow the eating regime outlined in chapter 22

Low Fat diet

This would seem to be a natural conclusion that if you have less fat in your diet you will lose weight, this is true, but only if you do it right.

If you reduce your fat intake too much, it can be harmful, because fat is not only visible on your body but it is also used as a cushion for the bodys organs & acts as a shock absorber.

If you don't reduce your fat intake enough you tend to gain weight & the excess fat gathers in unsightly rolls of flesh.

The secret of losing weight is to create an energy deficit by lowering your calorie intake, this generates an alarm signal in the brain which in turn instructs the body to start burning its reserves of body fat as a source of energy.
1 Gramme of fat contains 9 calories.
1Gramme of Alcohol contains 7 calories.
1 Gramme of Protein contains 4 calories.
1 Gramme of Carbohydrate contains 3.75 calories.

35—40% of Calorie intake per day in the U.K. comes from Fat.

To reduce & lose weight at a safe rate the ideal calorie intake should be 20—30 %, this is the recommendation of the W.L.R. (Weight Loss Resources).

Less than this recommendation is too restrictive & creates more problems than it solves.

Audrey Eyton,s famous "F" plan diet is considered by many experts to be one of the best balanced & achievable results programmes around.

As I said before this book is a guide to healthy living & not a specific diet book but there is enough information & guidance to establish a personal dietary routine that will help you achieve your goals whatever they may be.

EPILOGUE

I have endeavoured to write this book with as much relative expertise & integrity as lies within my scope of knowledge, also I have drawn on the expertise of other Professionals, Experts in their field, to substantiate my statements or opinions, I have also been quite blunt & very frank in places, primarily because I felt I had to be in order to emphasize the importance or gravity of a given situation, I have also felt it necessary to include some basic Anatomy & Physiology to illustrate the various body systems & how they operate both normally & in relation to Disease.

While the Medical profession have come in for some scrutiny,& criticism, especially those involved in the treatment of cancer this is not in any way intended to be a slight on the profession in general, indeed I myself was a Registered Nurse (Psychiatric) & also worked in General Hospitals & Nursing Homes & had a good rapport with a wide variety of Medical Professionals so I fully understand the pressures they work under, however I believe that the financial incentives offered to Doctors to promote the numerous types of Drugs & Vaccines plays a big part in their decision as to wether or not they should give their Patients **all** the facts about their treatment, knowing, as

I am quite sure many do that there are better & safer alternatives like the ones mentioned in this book, & for many Doctors, telling their patients the truth does indeed in the eyes of the Medical Higherarchy constitute a "revolutionary act".

Cancer, like many other diseases, can be deadly if not treated properly & with the appropriate treatment & I, along with other like minded health professionals firmly believe that many Cancer patients who have passed on would still be with us & also be healthy & Cancer free if the right treatment had been made available to them, alas, in the end many never even knew about "Alternative treatments", the ones that really work, that is, and so they never really had an informed choice of options let alone receive them, & in the vast majority of cases they have died from the Treatment rather than the disease, Remember **"Iatrogenic medicine"** in chapter 4?(most Doctors will not deny this) Many others live in constant fear & dread, hoping for a cure, not knowing that one has been available for the last 70 odd years, but you should know by now after reading this book that this need not be the case, there is more than enough relative information in this book to put you on the road to recovery & freedom from the fear of Cancer or any other Disease.

To those of you who struggle with Obesity & the craving for food, I am sympathetic, because I have also been Clinically Obese to a limited extent at various times in my life, especially since entering the middle age range, so I know how hard it is to lose excess weight, but I have done it, I pushed myself mentally & physically & I will not deny it was hard & many times I felt frustrated because it was not coming together quickly enough, but I persevered & am well on the way to getting where I really want to be, If I have seemed insensitive or abusive or insulting it has not been with bad intentions, indeed in many cases I have quoted the very same words the Bible uses, but you also have to understand the gravity of your situation both physically & spiritually, Jesus said "If you love me keep my commandments" Serving God requires sacrifices, Do what you feel you have to do to be what God wants you to be, & you will have the satisfaction of knowing you tried & were obedient.

I am persuaded also that just as the Children of Israel were rebellious & grieved God, modern day Believers are doing exactly the same & are reaping the consequences of their disobedience to his divine laws which were given for their health & wellbeing & I trust that this little book will in some measure ignite a flame that will be the catalyst for a Holy Ghost Fire that will spread around the World & enlighten believers & non believers alike & enable them to See & Feel & Know the benefits of healthy living gained through a knowledge of the Creators very own food laws, specifically designed to meet the demanding needs of life as we know it," Knowledge is Power" so do not let your life be "Destroyed for Lack of Knowledge", I have laid out for you the basics of healthy living as simply as I know how, If you wish to transform your life both Physically & Spiritually the Bible is the final authority in all matters of life & living.

GO FOR IT!!

Yours Sincerely,

Tom Pritchard.

BIBLIOGRAPHY

(1) See you at the top, Zig Ziglar (1983)

(2) European Human Rights Legislation (ECHR) 1998

(3) Journal of American Medicine (30/07/2000)

(4) Government Pesticides & Residues Committee 2007

(5) Richard Gunning R.T.U. Ministries.

(6) Alternative medicine Definitive guide to Cancer

Burton Goldberg 1997.

(7) Dr.Joseph Mercola (www.mercola.com)

(8) Dr.Joseph Mercola (www.mercola.com)

(9) Dr.Joseph Mercola (www.mercola.com)

(10) Philip Day - Health Wars (2002)

(11) Daily Mail (August 2007)

(12) Dr.Joseph Mercola (www.mercola.com)

(13) Dr.Joseph Mercola (www.mercola.com)

(14) Philip Day –Health Wars (2002)

(15) The coming of the saints (John w.Taylor 1969)

* ADD ABOUT

About the Author

ISBN 1425167780-2